JOURNEY INTO MY LIFE

I0104278

Lisa Diallo

chipmunkapublishing
the mental health publisher

Lisa Diallo

Published by
Chipmunkapublishing
PO Box 6872
Brentwood
Essex CM13 1ZT
United Kingdom

http://www.chipmunkapublishing.com

Edited by Kayla Pratt

Chipmunkapublishing gratefully acknowledge the
support of Arts Council England.

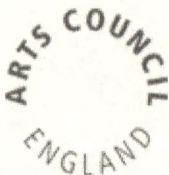

ARTS COUNCIL ENGLAND

Journey Into My Life

Chapter 1

1. State Of Mind
2. My World of Avoidance Disorder
3. Confusions And Delusions
4. State Of Mind Becomes Unkind
5. Mind Blowing
6. Grasping At Straws
7. Over The Edge
8. The Last Straw
9. Stay Strong
10. Fighting Back
11. Inner Strength
12. Don't Quit
13. You Guide Me Through
14. Divine Purpose
15. Island Of Freedom
16. A Way Out
17. Home Alone
18. Going It Alone
19. Another Chapter
20. Happy Birthday To Me
21. Get Back Up
22. Gone Too Soon
23. Happy Birthday Grandad
24. Faded Away
25. Remembering You're Gone
26. Passing Over
27. Forever With You
28. I Needed You
29. Never Forgotten
30. Oxygen Supply

Lisa Diallo

Journey Into My Life

State of Mind

Everyday always seems to be the same; I wake up
playing the same old game.
As one day just rolls into another, sometimes when
I wake I seem ok, then other I question why I bother

Same old routine, kids go to school, and then home
for a day of cleaning,
It may seem like I am moaning, but I am tired of the
same old feelings.
Health, for 3 out of the 4 siblings suffers with ADHD
and Autism aswell,
And nothing can make that better not even any
amount of wealth

I am so often told that life is what you make it,
I believe some people call it living,
But when you get no returns and it seems I am to
my children forever giving

For I am trying to understand myself with the help
of a C.P.N., but prescribed medication I cannot take
for the feelings that they give me, my strength it just
seems to break, and then I am not really sure how
much more borderline personality can or will take

For I know that obstacles are put in my way in life,
not just for me but I assume so many,
But to help myself and my children lead a normal
life, I would give every penny

Lisa Diallo

For this is how the routine goes, you're given your diagnosis followed by long medical words some you may recognise but most you have never heard, then you're given a psychologist there to sort out what's in your head, and here's your D.L.A. Each month, and all of a sudden you feel your existence is dead and so any pride you walked in with from you has all now been shed

And with all this you're expected to understand and you're supposed to know how to carry on,
When really your heads just blown away and all your rational thoughts have gone

And all those people you thought were friends have all slacked behind,
Looking for any reason for me to hide,
Because when the going gets tough as they usually do,
The only person that you can rely on "Is you"

For all I see, all deception and lies
Left paranoid in my own little world and for me the result became unkind
For I don't have many qualifications or even letters before my name
But between me and my four children I have mastered the health game

For Borderline Personality Disorder is something that only recently became recognised as coming under the Mental Health Act.

Journey Into My Life

But now all feelings of guilt and shame are all that's left for my mind to attack, and I know that there is no one else to blame,
Which makes me question if my mental avoidance can take any more pain

And everyday that I have survived and I'm still here to tell all truths of my past childhood abuse, and of drug misuse,
from teenage assaults to unlawful imprisonment, violence and mental torture, and believe me I know that these things hang around to haunt you

And all of this in just 34 years but I am still here fighting back.
Still overcoming my everyday fears
So the message that I am sending to all that have or still do suffer the way I do.
You need to know that you are stronger than most to survive this struggle they call life, and still manage to come through

For I have been as low as I can possibly go
To being pregnant and living in the streets,
Losing my home and my children and still taking my partners beatings.
So the only way I know is up, and I believe I am halfway there, as I have my home and my children back and if you want to know how I did it,

I believed in myself when no one else cared.

Dated: 30th July 2007

Lisa Diallo

My World of Avoidance Disorder

Feelings of loneliness is all that now fills my head,
Never to sleep or even just rest in my bed
Feelings of being unsure of what now fills the room
or even what lays behind the closed door,
For my imagination is now running wild, hearing
voices that are not really there, then repeated
memories of childhood dreams of searching the
streets to find my way home, and yet again I am
still alone for no presence it bares

Thoughts continuously going over in my mind
avoidance not allowing me any sleep to find,
And so the next day I shall be tired and weary,
Yet avoidance not allowing me to give in,
No it does not stop my concentration of thoughts
and feelings of insanity are all it has brought

And everyday is the same for me,
For I am lucky to be able to sleep, as soon as my
eyes awake from my dreams,
My thoughts my actions before me do leap,
Trying to concentrate on any small thing, but yet
again my mind wishes to explore, causing my
weary body to fall to the floor, for a clear mind is all
I now plead, I beg, I give in, as inside I scream

Rushing ahead of myself planning things for days
to come
And it then only brings me the chance to worry
about the things

Journey Into My Life

That have yet not happened, the things I have yet not done,
And although my brain wishes to do all these things,
To my body it only brings weariness,
Desperation and pain and so I find, never to recover from my minds own self harm

A lifetime of confusions, making anger all that's in control,
Lack of confidence and a big fear of change, and the biggest obstacle to get my head around is that there is no one else to blame, are the feelings I'm going insane

I can only describe at best it's like living in a foreign country, but you never learn the language,
No understanding of what people may say? And for people with Avoidance Disorder, this is something that I shall have to live with every single day.

Dated: 29 July 2004

Lisa Diallo

Confusions and Delusions

Confusions, Confusion
Is all that now fills my mind?
Trying to look to the future yet still keep falling
behind
All the realisations now I am seeing of how this life
can treat you
So cruel and unkind

Seems like I always lose something,
As I continue my search for something that cannot
be found
Feels like a winding road going around and around

Looking for happiness but still I cannot find
Or is it just this disorder and it's taking over my
mind.
Just longing for some love or even someone to be
kind

Then when I stop searching and my journey should
come to an end
I find that I am still alone
With not even one friend
No home calls to make and not even one text I can
send.
Here alone and I know that there's no one I can
blame as this mental disorder has taken over my
brain
Only to result in
'I feel I'm going insane'

Journey Into My Life

Then comes the realisation that everything I have been looking for
Was right here in front of my eyes
But the avoidance I pursued
I found to love I was blind
Denying how I truly feel telling myself that everything is bliss
When really emotions are now telling me that true love is
What I now miss

For the times that I sit with no sound
My mind searches for more
And the more my mind wants seems all shuts up tight like another closing door
My feelings all put on display as I can no longer hide
And still no response
So I guess once again my request was denied

And so reality kicks in
As disillusioned again I have been and all the results
Are as to others I became mean
For the feelings I have shown not wanting to be alone
Watching and waiting as my personality becomes cloned

And yet again it's too late as I know
'I've messed up'
All the tears I have shed and all hurt is now dead
And I know I shall have to remain strong in my head

11

Lisa Diallo

For I admit there is no one else to blame for all
feelings now become free
So optical illusions is now all that I see
Anger and Hate through my mental health
Has become the better of me.

Dated: 5th December 2005

Journey Into My Life

State of Mind Becomes Unkind

They say that my mental health is but a state of mind
Our illusions, confusions, and delusions I so often find
For the feelings that I'm losing control and that reality
I need to get a grip
Before my sanity has totally gone resulting in
Flipping my lid

But for me all has become a way of life
Not sure what is supposed to be normal anymore
For one minute I was so happy and the children and the whole family life
So proud to be someone's wife

Then in a matter of hours
Creeps in feelings of anger
Being alone, feeling frustrated and distraught
Leaving me to result in only anyone to fight
Grabbing the first thing in sight,
Scissors, plates, table or even a knife

And so when I have what I call an
'Explosion of the mind'
I know that I treat people so unkind
It's as if rage takes over, and my soul the devil does now define.

For like a volcano I just erupt,
God forbid

Lisa Diallo

The one who interrupts
For a sharp tongue, and a dangerous mind, is what
you shall find
And I question again why does my mental state of
mind become so unkind

For at times I can go too far
And I ask for all insight to stand clear
For I never know what I am capable of
Killing someone my biggest fear
For so often people take advantage of my kind
nature
And exploit my friendly ways
I wish they would realise how severely I am going
to have to make them pay

For they shall be made to pay for when my
explosions of the mind
Shall erupt for the final time
And no living person shall be left in my minds sight
For when I go
I shall take all those people and then maybe they
shall realise
How much pain they had put me through

For to play with my mind
You have to be brave or of the dangerous kind
For justification is something I never seek to find
And so I shall leave what remains far far behind
And then my stories shall be told
Of how my mental state of mind
'Then became so unkind'.

Dated: 1st July 2007

Journey Into My Life

Mind Blowing

Down Down Down
Like an everlasting fall
With echoes of an ever fading voice, for a faded noise
Is the only way I can explain my life
For the continuation and concentration in my life I have never known
Which results in being unhappy as every part of my life
'I've been disowned'
For my mind seems to condone the fears I have of
Forever being alone

There's a hundred and one things happening around me
My eyes, they see it all
Yet still inside my head feels like a fairground ride
Knowing eventually mentally I shall fall
Yet still trying hard to find a balance and to space everything out
Still trying to find a way to erase all my personal doubts
Still confusion within only allows me to scream and shout

And although my eyes see it all
My mind stores all that it sees inside
So even at those times when I feel like dying
My avoidance allows all the hurt to subside
Yes life masks my fears
Yet again I manage to hide

Lisa Diallo

Tick Tick Tick
Like clockwork everything goes
Like a second-hand of the ticking clock
And no one can possibly know if it shall ever stop
For eventually everything is destined to break down
For then is when it shall become silent
And shall no longer make that everyday sound

Like the technical divide we call our brain
Should ever become dysfunctional or for whatever reason
Should start to lose time
That is when it shall become clear for that is when they say
'You're about to lose your mind'

Just like a box big enough to fit in five things
Yet feels like someone has squeezed in ten
Feels like too many people in an already overcrowded room
Or two children in a very small den

Self combustion is now only left to remain
Your fears and anxieties, my mind blocks all pains
All is not allowed to be free, yes all released and let out
But not knowing who the one that shall lose
Who do I look for?

Which person mentally do I abuse?
For the person who witnessed the explosion of my mind
Shall no longer remain
To be able to tell my story of how to me

Journey Into My Life

This life became unkind

For closure of the heart, mind, body and soul
Then only becomes a secret
That no one shall ever unfold.

Dated: 1st June 2004

Lisa Diallo

Grasping at Straws

Grasping at straws has become a familiar part of my life
Trying to hold onto a family
And trying to be the best wife

Always searching and needing to feel
'Wanted and Loved'
Always wanting everyone to approve wondering whether to stay or make another move

Always hanging onto the last threads after my personality changes back
But only to heartache
For me now remains
For my borderline personality leaves me nothing to gain

Sometimes settling for second best
Just to avoid complications, trying to avoid landing myself into
'Yet another mess'

But there is always another thread that I can hold on to
Something to fall back on when everything goes wrong
Then the same as before
I am straight back looking for more
For somewhere to belong

Journey Into My Life

Wondering if I shall ever be loved and wanted by
anyone
By someone that loves me for me
Just left wondering if happiness I shall ever be.

Dated: 21st June 2006

Lisa Diallo

Over the Edge

Go on keep pushing me!
Till you can push me no more
Cause when that little something clicks, I'll take you
to the floor
Seems like your trying to see how much I can take
But what you don't realise is my front to you is all
fake
For I shall make you believe I am in control
Until the point where I can take no more

For that's the day when for you it shall end
And all the rules with you I shall bend
Because I shall take you to the floor
Then explosion of the mind I shall begin to explore
And then in my head you shall be no more

For when you mentally push me to the edge
You shall eat all those words that you once said
All those words when you thought you were clever
When you get an attitude your only response is
'Whatever'

For you're a little boy in a big mans world
For you are nothing for anyone to fear, and yet
You expect everyone to be sincere
You never listen to advice and you never adhere
So self punishment you brought upon yourself now
payback for you
Is all that can be dealt

So you're nearly there, yes nearly at the edge

Journey Into My Life

And still my patience you continue to test
And so all I can say is you've been such a fool for
you're the one who chose to
'Break the rules'
For when I reach that point and once too often you
messed with my head
That is when you have to realise your going to end
up dead.

Dated: 17th July 2007

Last Straw

Cracking up ready to give in
Even to kill and commit every sin, my head racing
Yet it feels like the brakes no longer work
Like the rage inside, it will no longer stop and so for
now all feelings and memories are to subside
Yes for now all seems to be forgotten

Now who is the one that dares to get in the way?
For I feel like a stick of dynamite slowly burning
away
Feelings of being scared of what the outcome shall
be
As red is for danger
And now that's all I see

Why? Why? Why?
Is all that circles my head
The thoughts of anger, revenge and suicide, am
starting to believe
I would be better off dead
For this thing they call life is full of shit
For it has offered me no happiness
No not one little bit

I have always believed that we are here to sit one
of Gods little tests
Just did not realise that it did not end until we are
laid to rest
So please can anyone answer me this
When did any test last 32 years all that is offered is

Journey Into My Life

Unemployment, violence only resulting in malice and tears

For this is not life or any set test
For this thing I call existence
One shall survive not evens life's best
So stuff what is right, stuff achievements, and defiantly stuff the law
Because up to you now
After all I have seen in this life
It has offered me nothing, no stuff at all.

Dated: 16th June 2004

Lisa Diallo

Stay Strong

There are times in this life when you may feel like giving in
And even sometimes feel like you are being punished for everyone else's sins

When everything you see is negative
All that surrounds your mind is doubts
Feeling inside that you are trapped by your fears, screaming
With long urges that you just want to get out

But just take a look back at the last time when you felt this way
When dark clouds are all that fills your days
Remembering all feelings of no way out
For its then you should remember the happiness that followed that
Came in several bouts

For these are just testing times
To see how strong we really are, to see if we can achieve this journey called life
To see how long we can cope and for how long and how far
So take heed of your inner self that still lays dormant within
Think of all those things that you have pulled through and maybe struggled with your feelings
But still remembering to give in

Stay strong until the end showing all around you

Journey Into My Life

That you can win this fight, remembering always
Never to quit
No not even one little bit
For these testing times shall be around for a while
so pick yourself up and get ready for the next mile.

Dated: 4th June 2005

Lisa Diallo

Fighting Back

Fighting back is what you must do
Even when the odds are stacked against you
Never listen to life's fears but continue to fight this
life with open ears
Listen to advice but have a decent say
Then tell them to go away
Think of number one and trust them not
They're best away
Yes all forgot

Because when you are young and naïve
Your looks and appearance do deceive
So when in life they jump on you, then there's only
one thing left to do

That's fight back against these make believers
Who love to smirk, grin, and tease
For they are just bullies who think maybe they are
the best
But really they are just here for our inner strength to
test

So stand up for yourself
Don't even contemplate walking away, just knock
them down
Don't preach or pray, for you know now this is the
only way
Yes it's time to make them bullies pay

For now you see

26

Journey Into My Life

It becomes a different fight and so it's time to convince others
That you are right
Now is not the time to worry about what has been said and done
Just hold your head high cause this is one fight you won't lose

So for my children and many others too
I hope these words inspire them
For if or when they should be faced with this situation
As I'm sure this life shall guarantee
Always believe in yourself
And admiration is all there for you to see.

Dated: 3rd July 2006

Lisa Diallo

Inner Strength

These things are sent to try us, is what someone
once did say
It's strange how some days are filled with sunshine
Yet others bring us on our knees to pray

But today these few words that I write are
especially for you
For the times when life seems dull and grey
And tears and sadness is all that fills your day

I wanted you to know that I am only a phone call
away
And that I shall always be here for you
For the bestest friend you have become
Your qualities just keep shining through and for
those reasons
I wanted you to know
I appreciate everything you do

I hurt when you are hurting
I get angry when you are sad and frustrated when
you are mad
And happy when you are glad
But every time I know that our friendship we have
Together shall defeat anything that is bad

For one of your finer qualities
Is the strength that you hold within
For you have come through so much
Considering everywhere that you have been
And I am so proud to have you

Journey Into My Life

'As a friend'
Yet I still hurt from the pain you have been living

So keep your head held high and your confidence strong
For I am never many miles away if you feel that you need somewhere to belong.

Dated: 1st December 2004

Lisa Diallo

Don't Quit

When things go wrong as they sometimes do
When the road you are trudging seems all uphill

When the funds are low and the debts are high and
on the outside you smile
Yet inside you long to cry
When all that caring is achieving is to get you down
a bit
Rest if you must for awhile but please promise
Not to give in
Don't quit

As success is a failure inside out
They are just life's thoughts of everyone's doubts
For you can never tell how close you really are
It may be near
Yet is seems so far

But please just remember one thing
That's to stick to the fight when you are hardest hit
For it's when things seem at their very worst
That you should not give in
There's no time to quit.

Dated: February 2004

Journey Into My Life

You Guide Me Through

You guide me through all my fears and worries and
all traumas in my life
For you guide me through my saddest times
Through all my doubts and strife

For when I am feeling low
And it feels like I don't belong and I have no where
to go
I feel your wings around me and as they do unfold
And once again a feeling that I belong
A secret shared and never to be told

The warmth you place around my heart brings me
comfort everyday
And then for all my up's and downs yet again on
you
I can rely
As I now know that you are the one person that for
me shall always be there
For your love is unconditional
And your nature is just to care

For you have helped me to see things clearly
Yes you became my sight
And when in certain situations with answers I battle
and fight
And when everything goes dark
You guide me through and bring me back out into
the light

For you are my guardian angel

Lisa Diallo

And you are with me everyday
Although some people do not believe and assume
my mind has gone astray
They do not feel the things you make me feel
For they are not open minded people
And for me it is all real
For everyday you protect me
And around my heart you place a seal.

Dated: 24th November 2006

Journey Into My Life

Divine Purpose

Searching......
For my divine purpose in life
Every single day
Yes
Searching yet still never seem to find
Looking for love and seeking all truths
Asking the questions if I shall find myself asking
'Shall I ever be loved again?'
I mean loved just for being me?
Who is going to be that special person that stays
around?
For the real me to see
And to allow my love to flow free

Tired of being alone
Although so many voices inside of my head
Then remembering all those other people who just
resulted in taking me to bed
But still for that one moment in time
That closeness of someone else it made me feel so
special
Yes so special that it almost seemed real

So my divine purpose said to be
A light worker as are the angels up above
Only difference is I work down here
Forever guided and protected by God and the
angels
So that I shall never experience any fear
But surely earth angels need somebody too
If only to talk away the pains of each day

Just someone to hold you and to say everything
shall be ok
And everything's going to be alright
And so just knowing someone's there when I turn
out the lights

For the part of my mission is that I always have the
comforting words to give that people need to hear
To make their lives have reason again
Bring happiness not tears
Filling peoples lives
Giving them a will to carry on
Make them see it's all worthwhile
And then for that moment in time, their worries and
fears shall be gone

So I ask
'Whom is it that offers these comforting words to
me?'
And for some reason I now need to hear like never
before
For who shows me to the guiding light
And who is it that opens all my future doors?

And I pray where my guardian angel is?
When I am feeling weak with my thoughts that I
cannot carry on
It's when the angels subconsciously picks me back
up as they know that I would never wish to be
without
Yet I still yearn for that physical love from another
earth person
And if I shall ever find I now start to doubt

Journey Into My Life

For it often feels like all of these things are in front
of me
Yet none of them offer me anything
And only when I await my transmission
Shall I no longer have this suffering?

Dated: 21st September 2006

Lisa Diallo

Island of Freedom

The island of nowhere I need to be free
Away from this grim harsh reality
Nowhere to run and nowhere to hide
Feels like I'm going out of my mind
So I take myself off to my special place
Just me, my radio and my island where I often go

For my island goes far into the distance
Way beyond anyone's sight where there is no
arguing, judgement and most of all fights
For the cruelty has been all taken out
Everyone's the same and yourself you never
question or doubt

Yet to return home remains in my thoughts
Thinking of all kinds of things
All problems still left for me to sort
But my island of freedom my worries it allows me to
abort
For me to change reality now becomes just another
mindless thought

So have to break free from this island of freedom
Every time I go home and I can arrive in style
For back there society makes you just a number
Then just added to the file

So for now allow your mind and soul to break away
And take you on a journey to some fictional place
For please do not let me return to that world of sin
For their lifestyle can break you

Journey Into My Life

And make you give up and give in

So I do wish I did not have to return to the island of
hell
For then how shall I ever have anymore stories to
tell.

Dated: 28th December 2002

Lisa Diallo

A Way Out

So much anger I feel inside
All my tears I still try to hide
Not knowing which way to turn and left forever
Wondering if me you shall find

The beatings everyday
The mental scars you did leave,
I know that no ones really interested still looking for
someone in me to believe

So in my house I lock myself away
And hope
That he does not return today
And I wish and pray for someone to help me, and I
pray that he will
Go away

Frightened for my daughter also fearful of my life
For what will it be next time?
His fist again or maybe this time a knife
I need someone to help me, before he takes our
lives

And then someone did hear my prayers
Maybe the lord did hear me
As the women's aid came
Rescued they took me in and gave me a chance to
be free

For they took me in and made me feel safe

Journey Into My Life

And it was such a joy again just to see my
daughter's smiling face
At last I had hope I could see a light ahead
And it was then that I realised
Happy without him I could be

But all my thanks to the women's refuge
For they were my guardian angels that day for they
rescued me
Before
He could return and make me pay
For all the tremendous support they gave me, not
just the workers
But also the other victims of violent abuse, they
gave me purpose showed me I could be of use

So if ever you should find yourself feeling trapped
and a prisoner in your own home
And you need someone to talk to who shall not
condone
Then every time the workers aid
Shall come first yes for me
They are the top of the list for they made me realise
That I am worth more than this violent abusers fist
They gave me a new life
A reason for me to carry on
And they gave me the confidence and strength to
make sure he was gone.

Dated: 10th January 1999

Lisa Diallo

Home Alone

Feelings of being insecure also feelings of being
alone
No one to talk to and as usual no one is answering
the phone
Feelings of no where to turn and again no where to
run
Only the hurtful memories that left me feeling numb

One month I have everything,
My husband my children
And a future worth reaching for
A great feeling of balancing on cloud nine
All hopes soared
Then in just the blink of an eye, all has gone
My husband
The secure family environment
That's what caused me to lose my will to carry on

Seems to be so unfair that to be given something
so good
Just for it to be taken all away
I realise it teaches us appreciation and learns us
how to survive
Only for us to get through another day of this
existence we call life

But now I question
How many times do we have to be shown?
How many times are we to learn about respect or
appreciation?
That we have accomplished many times before

Journey Into My Life

As eventually hearts will break
Causing lack of oxygen then physically fall to the floor
With no will power or strength to fight anymore

For I feel I have reached a point in my life
Where I don't want to experience all these things again
I don't want to sit anymore of life's tests
For I could go on forever searching for life's best

I believe out there, there is someone
And our mission in life is to find that one person
Made for us
And like everything else to get our dreams you know that as well as good
There shall be times that are rough

But for now I have decided to sit back for awhile
Maybe pretend for awhile to be in denial
And so if that person that is meant for me should ever seem to be around
Then here I shall sit waiting in the hope that I shall be found.

Lisa Diallo

Going it Alone

Single parents
That title so often condoned
People think the worst when you have kids and live alone
Comments are passed like
"She wants a father for her kids" or
Maybe it's that she's not doing well on the social money that they give

Or even that they just wanted council housing
Or even just enjoyed too many men
Seems they forget how to use protection, looks like she blames her parents
Claims she was never taught, or never had enough money so condoms
She could never have bought

All these things that are said to categorise everyone
Assuming everything for them is now gone
To assume they shall be a victim of the next boy's thoughts
Knowing quite well there is nothing she can be taught

Then I am left wondering
If anyone sits back and takes a look at how she really feels?
How did she ever get to this?
Maybe they think she has no feelings, she has been left with several kids

Journey Into My Life

Or maybe they just assume that she will never
survive
Maybe just maybe
She wants to become a wife

But all those people that sit in judgement
Know nothing of her life, no not one little bit
For here is a young girl going it alone
But she is still surviving and yes everything she's
got is all her own

Making ends meet just to stay off the streets
Not wanting to fail and result working in the beat
Now all these things she is doing just for her and
her kids
It's by far the most greatest qualification you shall
ever accomplish in this life.

Dated: 27th November 2004

Lisa Diallo

Another Chapter

Another chapter in my life
For my last resulted in me becoming a wife
But now another chapter I have to begin feels like
That amazing lover I felt
Was so very long ago
I just pray that this next chapter does not hold that
hurt through love anymore

Yes a new beginning a new cycle a chance for me
to start again
To start afresh
Try to rectify my previous mistakes
And make some good out of what turned into an
emotional mess
Yes I am ready to get back up
Time to carry on and continue this fight

For ahead are new challenges all ready to come
my way
Having to make that important decision
If you move on or remain strong and stay
Not knowing what is in store
Only this time I'm going forwards and behind me is
when I shall close the door

And for every door that I close, there's another one
being left ajar
With promising new horizons
With all chances that shall take me far
For me now everything lays ahead and in that I find
comfort

Journey Into My Life

As I retire to my bed

With feelings of being excited yet scared to awake
And find out what challenges shall first greet me
Question is will there be a new love
Or shall it be a single life completely?

Whichever way I am going I am sure I will survive
After all we are only given one chance at this precious life.

Dated: 6th September 2005

Lisa Diallo

Happy Birthday to Me

Happy Birthday to me, oh what a glee
Still cannot see the fun in becoming 33
Birthdays are definitely worse the older you get
But one thing I did not realise is that
They got morbid just yet

So the night before my birthday
I sit trying to find a friend
Or maybe just a hand to lend
Just to celebrate my birthday and now I'm about to give in
Surely this has to be a sin

So I decided to just sit and wait for my man
Surely he will cheer me up
And just when you think things could not get any worse
Guess what?
Another run of bad luck

As he has just arrived
To say he cannot stay
So now I'm feeling really shit
So can someone answer me
Why does everything keep going wrong?

So I guess no one to talk to
Not even one friend, not one who cares
And so it's at times like these that life really sucks
Cause at 33 my arse is still waiting on lady luck.

Journey Into My Life

Get Back Up

I sit today and write these words of inspiration
To remind me to carry on
Even when I feel like my whole world has been
turned upside down
And it seems like everyone I have ever loved is not
here
Or passed on

So I remember the last time
The last time when I felt like this
When my heart was broken and my soul was torn
to bits
And one thing I must now remember is never to
look back
Or even to feel sad at the things I had
For only on my heartstrings it shall attack
But I most remember to keep my mental state intact

For always to remember
What I had is now gone
Some of them good times that brought much
laughter
And fun
But eventually people and times change and you
must move on

And it's at that point that I realised
That they were just not meant to be
For the angels and my spirit guides
They knew there were better things that lay ahead
for me

So I just take hold of my memories
Of all that was shared
And just remember that I always did care
But my life's divine purpose has not yet been heard.

Dated: 3rd July 2007

Journey Into My Life

Gone Too Soon

Steven…
I will miss you now you have gone
Memories still flowing back from that tragic day
Memories of how it seemed so unfair
Too young I pray
Why was you not allowed to stay

As from babies we were brought up
Our baths we did share, our laughter, our tears
All taken for granted that these things would last
It only seems like yesterday
But for a short life lived
Now buried in the past
Steven you were too young to go
At just 18 your life should not have ended so fast

Even though no one shall ever take your place
Because Steven we both started out at first base
As you were my brother you was supposed to last
the pace
We shared the good and survived the bad
At them times big bro
You were all I ever had

As brothers and sisters go
I would say we were the very close
Remembering all those times
We went camping and all the secrets that we
shared
Things only me and you shall ever know
We promised not to tell

Lisa Diallo

Promised to take to the grave
But I did not mean right now and so much anger I
have
Inside all questions trying to get out
Why? Oh why? Why?

So young, so free, why you and not me?
All questions
But the answers now I shall never find
So please God answer
Why is life so unkind?
And everyday that we grew the more and more I
admired you
Yes you were the biggest part of my life
Always holding that special place deep down in my
heart
And that shall still remain the same
And even though I am sad that you're gone
Really you have just stepped into the next room
As when the angels came down your soul from
your body
With that they did swoon

So now you have laid your head to rest
And closed those sad yet young eyes
You are loved more than ever and shall be missed
even more
As at just 18 still seems so wrong to have to say
our last goodbyes.

Dated: May 2002

Journey Into My Life

Happy Birthday Grandad

Well another year gone by
It's almost eight years now since you passed
And thoughts and memories of you are still what fill
my days
So many times I try and talk to you
But the hurt still remains
Like the day you had to go
Oh Grandad
I miss you
So much more than you could ever know
I hope you can see that it still shows

Today should be a happy one
As another year older you would have become
But please forgive me grandad
But I cannot find the fun, and I know that you see
and hear me
Every single day
I think the hurt and the pain of losing you
Is definitely here to stay

Still cannot really accept that you had to go
Always thought you would be around forever
And still til this day
Hollins Road I cannot bear to go
For 605 shall for me
Never be the same again

Still hiding from the reality of it all
As the last time that I left that house
Was the day you left too

Lisa Diallo

In a horse and glass carriage I remained right
behind you
Hurting inside from the pain grandma felt
Wishing I could make things for her better
As for her the worst deal had been dealt

And every time I see her
The pain in her face does show
And seeing her alone is not the same
So I promised myself not to make the same
mistakes that I did with you
Like taking for granted you would always be there
I promised myself that for grandma
I would always remind her how much I cared.

Journey Into My Life

Faded Away

I write these words today
As I feel at this point in my life grandad it seems I
need you again
And I know the last few words I wrote for you
Started exactly the same
So now I have come to realise that without you
I have nothing left to gain

Even though you have passed away
I always used to feel you close
Beside me
Just the warmth that I would feel
Of you next to me
Or even the tightness when you held my hand
But now your aura is nowhere to be found

First your picture was to fade
Then the locket let loose from my chain
I pray tell me why did you let go?
And am I the one to blame?
For all that I am left with is this guessing game
Maybe you thought now a husband I have found
That somehow I would not need you around
Or that somehow you were not needed
But grandad
The only way that I survive is the thought of you
here
All the memories of you are still needed

For there shall never be a point when I will not want
you around

Lisa Diallo

For you
You were and still are the only one I could trust and believe in
For whatever wrongs I ever did or whatever sin I did commit
You always remained beside me in everything I did
You never disowned me, you never got rid

I don't understand
Why when at the most important time in my life
Like now when I feel like mentally giving in
Feels like I can take no more
It is at times like this I wish I had you here
Beside me
Whispering those comforting words that I did adore

Right now it feels like…
It feels like life is so unkind
Why did you have to go away?
Why did our Lord choose you?
For you were one of those better people that our world shall always need
And for fact I need you more
What did I do wrong in a previous life
For it seems that every time someone loves me
It then gets taken away
I wish I had the answers to what I did wrong and why I am being made to pay

So grandad
Even though your picture has faded
You're forever in my head
And that is the only thing that no one can take away
And until the day that we meet again

Journey Into My Life

That is where
Forever
You shall stay.

Dated: 11th August 2004

Lisa Diallo

Remembering You're Gone

How do I get through?
To get through life without you
I really do not know how I continue to survive
As you are the one and only person on whom I
could always rely
And still now since you're gone I somehow lost the
will to survive
As the roots were pulled out of my life
As you were my inspiration as with everything
You did help me get by

And still remembering how to love myself
That was a valuable piece of advice that you once
dealt
For you took the time to understand me
And fell the pain I had felt
Yet finding it hard to love all the things about me
That you could always somehow always see
You looked right into my soul and saw all
Saw all the pain and miseries that self punishment
had brought me

I have never felt so alone as I do today
And I have always and will forever feel that a part of
me died too
For everything I say
And everything that I do now
Is just little things now left to remind me of you

For you were the one that found good in me
And a trustworthy person you made me feel
Never criticised what I had done

Journey Into My Life

Never made me feel I did not belong
But most of all you showed love, admiration and in my eyes
You were always strong
You had the strength to see us both through
And never once complained and I guess that's why I never noticed
That your time was finally through and you were slowly slipping away

Yet still to this day
That is something you are remembered for
That you got through all the hurts and pains on your own
Never once did I hear you complain or moan
And for all that I honoured everything that you did
As you turned me into what I am today
A woman you raised in me from just a child

I just wish that this one time
You had trusted me and relied on me
To tell me it was time for you to let go
And then every last minute I would have saved for me and you
As I owed you at least that much
As you were my eyes when I could not see
And my mind taught me to set free
And you convinced me that I could be everything I wanted to be
And that everything I could get through
But one thing you forgot to prepare me for was
The day I lost you.

Dated: 23rd February 2005

Lisa Diallo

Passing Over

My grandad did not have a lot
But for all his children and grandchildren
He gave them all he got

47 years of marriage never to be forgot
All those precious years
Many children they did bear
And to them he gave the lot
Everyone was treated equally as my grandad was
always fair
As no matter what mistakes we did make
And a few I did make
He always had those special words
That reminded us that he still loved you

With all the pain he went through
And no matter what was wrong on his face a smile
Would always remain
Not only loved by his family, his friends all loved
him too
Just walking down Hollins Road everyone he knew
Always gave them the time of day
To stop and chat a few kind words as pulling down
his flat cap
He left a smile on everyone's face
Then he would call in the bookies and put a bet on
the next race

He never asked or expected much out of life
But love he always gave, his smile, his laugh, the
memories

Journey Into My Life

Are all now left for us to remain?
For these are what was made to keep us close and
forever safe
For now to a better place he has gone
Knowing that he shall be looking down on us all
and still smile
For in our hearts forever
And now no longer shall be tired

So even though we are left grieving and rivers of
tears we shall shed
Through the path of righteousness grandad you
shall now be led
For grandad we shall all miss you
As you had to go away
But there's one thing I never got chance to say…
'Goodbye and I shall love you always'

For the 15th of November 1998
Is a day I shall never forget
For that is when you passed over and laid your
head to rest
And even though it hurts so much
I know it is the right thing
As Grandad you always knew best.

Dated: 16th November 1998

Forever With You

Although Grandad you have only stepped into the
next room
Without you here my life has too much room
Although in my heart
Forever is where you shall remain
It doesn't stop the hurting and it doesn't stop the
pain

As when they made you grandad
They definitely broke the mould
As everyone you did meet, their hearts you did
unfold
My heart especially as you reached down deep
Now you're gone my heart skips a beat

So many things I wish I had told you when you
were alive
I wish I had held you more than I did
And now it is much too late as they sealed the
coffin lid
For the world has now lost one more, better person
Yes grandad that was you

And so now to a better place you have gone
As your work on this earth is finally done
Yes your struggle is over
And you achieved all that needed to be done
And for the times we shared together
All the memories are mine now that you're gone

So grandad, now go to sleep

Journey Into My Life

And rest in peace
Because in my heart you shall forever live on
And it's there I shall keep you forever
A comfort to me then you shall never be gone.

Dated: 3rd April 1999

I Needed You

I write these words today
As I feel at this point in my life that grandad
I need you more than I have ever needed you before
It is at times like these that no matter what the problem
Somehow you always gave me an inner strength
That helped me survive even more

Although I know that you are forever by my side
As your aura I feel all around
Yes those little signs letting me know that you are there
As the picture in my locket you reveal
Reminding me of how you always cared
Your smiling face is then what I see
And at that point I realised
That you was just letting me know that you are here with me

And yet even though you have been sleeping for some time
I often pray that somehow you will walk through that door
With that crazy smile you always held, that so often made me laugh
And again without saying a single word
I feel the love for me you always had

Your eyes so often spoke to me
All the pains and the joys I saw

Journey Into My Life

And those visions are forever in my heart and head
So even though you went to sleep
The memories are to forever remain
Which gives me hope that all is not dead

I wish sometimes that you could come to me
If only in my dreams
For it would fill me with so much hope
And maybe restore some faith that I lost the day
you left
And also I hope to give me a reason in this life to
believe
For grandad you were my strength
You taught me how to accomplish every self need

I know that it may seem that I am asking a lot
And anxious I become
The reasons being that I feel so many things where
left unsaid
For so many things were left undone
I do not expect for the answers to survive this life
Or even to tell me where I am going wrong
But just to know that you are watching over me
Gives me the feeling that somewhere I still belong

For you have always and always will be
The only man that remained in my life through thick
and thin
And that I trusted one hundred percent
This is why my heart still grieves from the pain of
losing you
And I fear I shall never be free
For you became my world
You meant everything to me

Lisa Diallo

And although I do not talk aloud anymore
I know that you sense when thoughts of you enter
my head
And they are for me alone
No one can share them; no one can take them
away
For they are mine alone until my dying day.

Dated: 14th April 2004

Journey Into My Life

Never Forgotten

Even though it has been five years now since you
decided to let go
These next few words that I write
Are just some of the things I wanted you to know?
My heart still aches, my eyes still cry
For when you decided to let go
I feel that with you a part of me also went with you
And so the pain I still feel
I still cannot hide

After those things in life threw at you
Now leaves me wondering
How did you manage to get through?
As since a child I remember I always relied on you,
For you were the father I never did have
You wiped my tears, took away my childhood fears
And always made me happy when I was feeling
sad and blue
For you're feelings you always kept inside
So very deep
And although you were always strong
I did not realise you had given up
And decided to go to sleep

Sometimes it feels like I have forgotten how to
grieve
As my eyes no longer swell
Yet still there lays a big space in my heart that you
did always dwell
Everyday I feel you beside me
In my mind, body and soul

Lisa Diallo

I seemed to have built my whole life around you
and made you my goal

Everyday I always have a thought for you
You just seem to pop inside my head
And so I wondered then if you see all the things
that I do
And that it gives me the inner strength
That I got from you
All I ever wanted was for you to be proud of me
And show everybody else
They were so very wrong
As even when you're soul did depart
My love and respect for you shall forever live on

Your stories of old we often heard
How many times used to be for you
Seems that things were not that easy but with what
you had
You had to make do
Never handed anything on a silver platter
You worked for everything you had
Bringing all you're strengths to survive
All good and bad
And so it leaves me wondering who was there for
you
For you had no one to catch you when you fell
Unanswered questions I guess
These are the stories you never did get to tell.

Dated: May 2004

Journey Into My Life

Oxygen Supply

Every breath I shall take I shall remember you
And every dream that I dream
Is now what sees me through
And every waking day that I get through
I wanted you to know my heart and memories
forever belong from you

For all the up's and downs life did send you
For all the sorrows and sadness that I somehow
caused
And for everyday that I took you for granted
And every minute that I did not appreciate you
For all those tears alone we did cry
From everyone else managed to hide
And now it's too late to say I am sorry
Without you I have lost my oxygen supply

And for all these things
Forever in my memory they shall stay
As we had to say our last goodbyes
Now making it my mission without you to survive
As even though I am happy that you are resting in
peace
Feels like someone tore out my soul
And now no oxygen is left to release

So even though I continue on this earth to exist
You're loving ways and toothless smile
Is just a few things that I shall forever miss
Yet always I shall know that through every bad
experience

Lisa Diallo

I shall ever come across, and every disappointment
that I am dealt
And it's a comfort to know that you're beside me all
the way
And then just a maybe
My oxygen supply should last for another day

Now memories we are given are made to last
Even if some of them took us into bad past
For they are reminders of the mistakes we have
made
And all the guilt felt was put there for us to pay
And from them a lesson we should of learnt
From the experiences of our fears for when you left
me grandad
It felt like over you I cried a river full of tears

So no matter what still happens
You were and still are
The only male in my life that made such a big
impression
But now the loss of your love and trust teaches me
of depression
For what I did not realise is that you were in control
of my oxygen supply
Leaving me for a failure to breathe as part of me
was lost
On November 15th 1998
The saddest of my whole entire life
Yes grandad it was the day you died

Grandad I still miss you so much
And I wait for the day that we shall meet
So please leave those pearly gates open wide.

Journey Into My Life

Chapter 2

Lisa Diallo

a Life

Oh what a life it has been so far
Time passes so quickly
So much of this life I have seen
It started so many years ago
Yes this thing called life gave me my get up and go

Yes it taught me to move around and travel
Yes many towns and cities
Listening to their talk, oh how some did waffle
At least I have had a life like a circus show
Experience has taught me everything I know
Everything I know, forever getting up to go

So much to tell the up and coming
All boils down to taking and giving
Just like the way it is turning out right now
Still searching for the light at the end of that tunnel
And it's nowhere in sight
It has to be somewhere out there

There are so many different people to meet
So don't sit about being lazy, get up onto your feet
And then go out there still soldering onto hope
That your life should never go wrong

You meet so many people in their own little worlds
It broadens your horizons
And you start to realise how little you really knew
Different faces and different places every kind for
you to meet
Now I am feeling lucky

Journey Into My Life

I think I may have landed on my feet

Oh no it's a figment of my imagination
The real parts I forgot
But be good if it has turned out nice
So if you're now thinking of moving away
Maybe after this you may think twice.

Dated: 1st Jan 2003

Lisa Diallo

The Streets

The streets of the city life go on talking
To some old faces
Then to the dole to sign on, no fixed abode, no
address
As the streets just go on and on

Talking to friends about who you saw last
Knowing that they are thinking you are a total bore
Going around in gangs thinking it is cool
Thinking they are macho when really they just look
like fools

For it's a boring life on the streets
Cities and towns
They are all the same
And everywhere I go to I question
Who for this life is the one to blame?
Because this life living on the streets
It's just a mugs game

Everywhere has its local crowd of people
Some are ignorant and some are not
And as usual there are a few that seem ok
But you never witness anything different
Still going round in circles every single day

The only thing left for me to say
Why is it that so many people are self inflicted?
Mostly its drugs
They have become addicted
Then they expect sympathy

Journey Into My Life

As they then become the victim

Addiction to drugs
It's not a question
Violence and prostitution is all that seems to remain
For life on the streets is no life
No there is nothing
There's nothing here to gain.

Dated: 27th December 2002

Lisa Diallo

The Point of Life

Does anybody really know what they want from this
life?
Is it a husband or a wife?
Do they want it easy or do they enjoy the struggle
and fight?
There are so many roads to take
Some lead to happiness whilst others lead to
sorrow
Some lead to the path that is right
And at the end of the path you have a choice
Turn away or step into the light

One day we are born and one day we will die
What's in the middle is up to you to make right
But what's in between you choose yourself
May it feel like heaven, or may it be like hell
No one can live their life perfectly and never make
mistakes
People always get hurt and forever hearts shall
break

But the secret of this life is
Live for today and not for tomorrow
Think of only happiness and discard any past
sorrow
The mistakes you have made try to put them right
Be happy of the days and be grateful of the nights
Never look back
Just reach out for what's in sight.

Dated: 29th May 2002

Journey Into My Life

Silenced Screams

One Friday night all alone
Sitting in my room
Paperwork everywhere, nothing exciting just all bills
and doom and gloom
When all of a sudden my silence was broken with
sounds of running feet
And then followed by many more as I remembered
The loud thudding beat

And that was when I heard it; it was the cries
Of a young man almost even a boy
A cry like no other I had heard before
"Leave me alone" he cried "I can't take anymore"
"No More" he begged
That's when the other footsteps stopped to a halt
There were several of them at a guess
And still the young man pleaded
That they stop this awful mess

Then several voices all spoke at once
So muffled I struggled to hear
And it was at that point this poor lad's life I did fear
Sat there all alone not knowing what he was going
through
But to attract attention to myself is something I
could not afford to do
Left with feelings of being helpless that I could not
make him safe
When all he really needed was a hiding place

Not sure what happened next or how it did all end

Lisa Diallo

As the streets once again became silent
And there was no one to be found
And so now the only thoughts that run through my
head was
How did they silence that man's sounds?

So as I lay my head to sleep
I hope and pray that God shall make him safe
And so those other thugs stop the chase
For the death of a young man no one should have
to face
Just because he was at the wrong time at the
wrong place
And so this story today just proves to me now how
our society
Has become a social disgrace.

Dated: 14th January 2006

Journey Into My Life

The Force

Tit tit tit
Here the engine through the night
Watch out here come the coppers torches shining light
Now hello hello died long ago
Now its just arm up your back
And in the van they then do throw

Don't need a barrier for a stopper
As stuck up your bum are several coppers
Not just one two or three
They travel in herds for you to see
Yet when you're in trouble they are nowhere to be seen
Yes all back to the station drinking tea

Yet when they are all out in their riot vans
And uniforms along with hat and truncheons too
Because as usual they are wasting time as they have nothing better to do
Then they come and arrest you as they please
And then throw you in the cells with the fleas

And yet again they have nicked you for sod all
At this rate you'll be entitled to tickets for the Christmas ball
And then they question you even though they know
You'll get the blame and then to court you'll go my son
Laugh out loud this is their idea of fun

Lisa Diallo

So now let the court case continue
To proceed you get a fine but there's no need
As straight away you walk away knowing that the
fine you'll never pay
So go ahead enjoy the sea and sand
Because you know the next time you're caught
You're definitely on remand.

Dated: 28th December 2002

Journey Into My Life

The Prisoner

Welcome!
Welcome to the prison says the prisoner with a long drawn face
Whilst smoking a match thin roll up
His only interest in his book he never lifts up his head unless
He wants to give you another of his dirty looks

The prisoner comes in on his own
And like all the others he is cloned
As he walks down the landing like he thinks it's his kingdom
But I don't think he's yet realised that he has just lost his freedom

Always plotting
Something up his sleeve
And always on the want or need
Like a hunter in the night
Yes the new prisoner prowls around just looking for a fight

With his prison mates they all gather round
And he sees them as his only escape
The walls are thin and you hear everything
Every little sound
And then their screams of pain eventually die down

The prisoner needs others to feel secure
Only feels safe behind closed doors
Because one man on his own may find

Lisa Diallo

The jail itself shall take over his mind.

Dated: 5th December 2002

Journey Into My Life

Who Needs Your Sort

You loud pratt
You get on my nerves
Attention you're seeking you travel in herds
Give me peace and quiet you freak
No wonder I'm finding it hard to hear myself speak

Your friends you seem to hide behind
You're never on your own
You're boasting and your loudness
It's all a front; yes yet again you're putting on that act
Now that is a fact not fiction
I believe you're lacking a sense of tact

You think you're hard and that's a shame
Just because you have letters before your name
And so you think you have experienced this thing called life
But have you ever had to use your fists in a fight?

So what happened when you were young?
Did something go terribly wrong as you're
pretending that your mind is strong
Who are you when you rob your friends
You low life scum
Then you smile to their face like you're having fun

In a prison or a hostel I would like to see your type
To see you would never make it through
You feed your addiction by feeding off others
Then when you have finished

Lisa Diallo

Yes you have had your fix
You always need another.

Dated: 4th December 2002

Journey Into My Life

Dimwit Dad

So! Why do I put up with this useless stepdad?
He's even worse than the others I have had
God when I have left here I shall be so glad
As then I don't have to worry about a miserable stepdad
Who is happy as Larry oh so great
When actually he looks like he has been slapped about the face
No conversations
No get up and go
All he does is repeat what he has told you five minutes ago

TV shops and a pot of tea
Pair of checked slippers and brain cells only three
All split into different parts
One shops one watches TV and three constantly think of playing darts
When he dies I wonder where he will go?
Maybe into another life
Maybe with a rainbow full of pretty colours, all mixed into one
Or with any luck maybe he shall turn into one of the puppets on the TV sitcom

With the brains of bungle and the body of George
Surrounded by fags, TV and food to gorge
For his clueless thoughts are gaps to be bridged
As his stomach alone contains half the fridge
Drop him from an aeroplane heading for the coast of Spain

Or even drop him in the sea
Only problem being is how to peel him off the settee

As then he shall call for help wishing his settee was his boat
And then I would push him out to sea
For I know that he would still have hold of the TV remote
He is an embarrassment to all my mates
And makes me feel squeamish if he should ever see my dates
And at my cost this I have found
Those mates and dates no longer do I see

So when he is told of what he has actually achieved
Casing his step-children to leave
But does he realise they left because of what he lacks
He has no life and that's a fact.

Dated: January 2000

Journey Into My Life

England

So welcome to this country of sin
With all the talk about everything they win
For you hear the blokes say
Let's go pull a few birds then go down to the pub
Suggests the fat English man who lives for his grub

No characters are in this jumped up place
For they never tell you straight to your face
And then we have the red white and blue football fan
He starts to kick off his excuse "because he can"
What he really means is his team has just lost
Yes just gone down the pan

Then there are others that feel they are unique
And they think they are like no other
But the truth be known when it all comes on top
They just go call big brother
And it's then I'm left questioning why people live in this way
Worrying about maybe when instead they should be worrying about things day to day

Whilst some buy a house with a mortgage
Along with a family and a dog and the two cars
Digging themselves just deeper into strife
Yes deeper in debt yet still they find time to comment
On other peoples life

And when the boredom eventually sets in

Lisa Diallo

The English few they precede to bullying and to fights
And it doesn't matter who or why
Just anyone who comes into sight

Whilst others are laid back
Just telling their stories to friends and other peoples wives
And all they can talk about is that they are living the high life
For these are snobby people in their soulless towns
Not aware of the reality that's around

So if you should ever visit England
Please do not be surprised if you have to take one step down
For all walks of life can be found.

Dated: ?

Journey Into My Life

Slave Labour

Don't let them make you work
Just pleasantly pass a grin or even a smirk
Employment for what who or why?
Packing boxes
No thanks would rather die

Or packing warehouse manual labour
Wear a hair net do me a favour
So what is the worst that can happen?
Oh no you could be fired
Oh well at least it gets your employer off your back

Employment you must be nuts
Working for a pittance and having to get up
A factory worker, miserable again and foreman saying what's your game

Then there are the moaning grannies with equal rights
And too many points of view, the working class ones are the best
Their hair, their teeth, oh what a mess

Like herds of cattle hear them groan
Oh someone pass that granny a bone
Tattooed women who are defiantly butch
I find their masculinity far too much
So do your best to stay unemployed
Don't go near work, please avoid
So just tell them you're tired
One bonus is then you cannot get fired.

Lisa Diallo

Fitness

So you think you're in control of your body and mind
There's something out there new to find
If you sit and slouch and give in
That will lead you to only lose and not win

Get up get fit today
And then beat the slob you portray
Lift those weights, get in the mood
Don't sit around moping and feeling blue

One week you will feel the ache
But please don't give up for God's sake
The more you go the better you will feel
It will make you sweat, squirm and squeal

In three weeks you won't regret
And you will be ready for another set
Fitness levels rise and your body changing
The last affect is amazing
Just like a car your engine running
You go through excruciating pain
So don't just sit there you only have yourself to blame

A boost for your mind and self esteem
So come on and join the fitness regime.

Dated: 28th December 2002

Journey Into My Life

No Character

No character is your name
Everything you do everything you say
Never say or do anything different
Everyday you speak the same
The same old moping face that you wear everyday
Looks like you were slapped at birth right in your
face

Oh what an interesting person you are
For only one brain cell, never got you far
You make me lose the will to live
You always depress me, something has to give
Go on try something new

Predictable is what you have now become
You're the one that climbs up that old age tree
But to me you always come and go
And then go and tell me all over again something I
already know

You go to work everyday without fail
Take that key out of your back as you're starting to
go stale
You wear the same thoughts all the time
So what gives you stamina
Yourself, you are still looking to find.

Dated: 6th December 2002

Lisa Diallo

Nightclub Girlies

Try to talk to them and you shall be ignored
With evil looks
And in your face they will shut the door
And then they turn to look and sweep back their
hair
Think the response is that I'm supposed to care

For these nightclub girlies they have foul mouths
And their hair scraggly bleached blonde
But really the roots are showing brown
They pass the guys and squeeze all bits
And then drink their beer
Then somehow they think they look hard
And everyone should of them fear

Nightclub girlies for years I have tried to make
some sense
But on the blondes I gave up as they are just too
dense
But on average they are usually fat and ugly things
Kind of like something the cat dragged in
God only knows what diseases they have
I dread to think where they have been

And it seems that the younger ones are the worst
Their clothes so tight they are bound to burst
For the last weeks man never stuck around
But that's no problem for these nightclub girlies
As soon another victim they have found

For when they are drunk they spit and slobber

Journey Into My Life

Bobble and weave
With their pit bull looks you're bound to heave
And it looks like some of these young girls are ten
years out of date
God should of left them at the devils gate
And God only knows where they came from
If they were hatched or found
But one thing is for sure these ugly girls are
nightclub bound

For so often their underwear meets their feet
Or they just carry them in their handbags
So everyone can clearly see
Tempers like a nuclear bomb; God only knows
where they came from
Or if to anyone they ever belonged

I personally believe they should all be caged away
So the rest of us can have a decent day
Or even better still send them to the moon
On an extremely large rocket
Go up and up as far as they can
Then stop!
Turn around and then just drop it.

Dated: 19th August 2005

Lisa Diallo

Students

Where the hell did they come from?
God only knows what drugs they are on
All their talk about boyfriends
Training to be a lawyer or even a scientist
And they believe that this is bliss
Not knowing of reality never having to struggle
Never having to use their fists

Seems that the female gender spends her life trying
to get her kicks
Whether it be going out clubbing
And all that is achieved is that she has collected
many pricks
And then when they finally meet the right man
They just bleed him dry for all they can

Always telling those crap jokes that we never get
Old fashioned clothes and the stains of sweat
Trying to work out what is the purpose of life
For now only education for them is rife
Wondering what the purpose is really for
Do they not know, in reality there is nothing at all

I'm sick of students everywhere you go
Who have boyfriends or girlfriends
In not one two or three, but six
Always looking for the next victim
That will supply their next fix
If I had my way I would hire a large bus
And drive them into the ground until they are dust.

Dated: 6th April 2005

92

Journey Into My Life

Male Species

The rubbish food they eat
And they push you about with their threats to beat
The looks they give you, like you are crazy
And then they come back with I love you
And will you have my baby

Selfish species they think they are the best
But when you've had one you've had the rest
It's me and it's my life say them all
As they sit back and watch, expecting you to fall

So why is it they cannot keep their big mouths shut?
And I got news for you
I don't give a shit about your judgemental looks
For they think they are big and strong
God you are so sad and again so very wrong

For you live your life like it is the Wild West
Giving your orders and setting tests
You can't cook or clean, because you say you can't be bothered
Your stale beer breath is now all that hovers

Then when it comes down to money
They take every last penny
And in return they think sex is a fair exchange
When all it means is washing the sheets and that's a pain
For I think that a mans mentality is the same as a wooden brush

Lisa Diallo

Thick wooden handle, yes cheap and tacky
Just waiting to bust

Lying, cheating, deception, more lies
Their immaturity makes them act like spoilt brats
For never speaking an honest word and they still
believe they are the best
But as many others before, they are shit
Just like all the rest.

Dated: 18th April 2005

Journey Into My Life

Life

It's cold and damp and it's starting to snow
And no one seems to care or even wants to know
And then the moment you start to pick yourself up
Then down you go and surprised you're stuck in another rut

So why is this life so painful to live
As seems we live it for nothing for none of its gains are ever shown
All there is, is the harsh realities
And to expect the unknown

In this evil life your patience may wear thin
For there's illnesses, disease they all start to set in
Life without arrogance greed and money
Would surely be painless safe but yet not funny

To go through proving to people that you are mentally strong
Not weak or feeble, trying to climb the ladder again
And get people to notice your fame
And when all is done and dusted, you think you have finally won
You turn a new corner then out of the blue
It turns itself around and it comes back to you

So it's back to life's dungeons of doom and gloom
I am needing some space maybe in another room
The perils of life's pressure, the pain of going round in circles
Just playing the game

So on and on the story goes
Where your life is heading, nobody knows
The condition of their health begins to show
Surprise surprise there is no more dice for you to throw.

Dated: 3rd December 2002

Journey Into My Life

My Unborn Child

First the news you're pregnant
Yes a child's on the way
The worry and the anguish that is brought with everyday
Everything is running smoothly hear the doctors say
Then comes the problems
And it's then you know that one way or another
Your heart is destined to break

From one day to another each little thing occurs
But as long as this baby is apart of me
My love is what we shall share
After all the problems we have been through
I long for that tiny cry from long ago
That baby's cry that I was never given the chance to know

That cry from yet so long ago
The child I never bore, the baby I so longed for
No longer exists is gone and no more
And now another chance I have been given
But I have already grown attached
I hope and pray that it is the healthy
As my feelings have already latched

And after all work is done and this baby is in my arms
I will forget about the pain and the sorrow
And concentrate on making sure he comes to no harm

Lisa Diallo

And then I suppose my bit for Britain is finally done
As now I am the proud mother of three beautiful
sons.

Dated: August 1994

Journey Into My Life

Love I Lost

I have three sons who I am proud of in each
individual way
But I still miss the hearty laughs since they went
away
As there is not a day goes by that I do not think of
you all
As my heart is torn in two
From the loss of my three little boys

I miss their laughs and their giggles
And even miss the sounds of your cries
And remembering these things just returns bad
memories
Of all the deceit and the lies
And so here I write the memories I will forever hold
of you all

Daniel you are the eldest
And already you have been through so much
And forever I shall be proud of you and shall always
long
For your hand to touch
As without you beside me in all the years gone by
Without you I would have never survived because
you became my oxygen supply
And most of all my life, and all I ever wanted was
happiness for you
And letting you go was my biggest sacrifice

Christopher I guess you are four now, not quite a
baby anymore

Lisa Diallo

And for what it's worth my heart is torn
For everyday I love you more and more
And I imagine how you are growing up, missing all
those things I used to adore
And I shall never be able to explain to you why I am
not around
To watch you as you grow up and help you through
life's tests
But I need you to know that no matter what you do
in life
To me you shall always be the best

Jordan last but not least, my baby
For you are still two and everyday that I live I shall
suffer only hurt and guilt
For I shall never have the chance to enjoy all the
love
In such a short time we had built
I never meant to hurt you but I guess your
innocence shall be a blessing
As it shall make you unaware of all that's causing
peoples hurt

And forever you shall remain in my heart
And my only hope is that one day for me you will
search
And replace that missing part of my heart
I guess the only words that I can say to you now
And these words are for when you are older
Is that somehow in this life I lost my way
And forever now it shall remain the fact I lost you
Everyday I shall be made to pay

Journey Into My Life

Although you may all feel like your lives have been
turned upside down
And may wonder why I let you go
I did it for your happiness, and I am still sat here
suffering the blows
I know I made the right choice now
As I could never give you all those things you
deserve
As for you all, all I ever wanted was the best
And I have realised that I failed you all
Yes I failed this thing called life's survival test

So I dedicate these words to you, my three little
boys
And although it was kinder to let you go
All the memories remain
And that shall be my eternal pain
But I hope as you get older you shall look back at
these words
And that they shall bring some comfort to you all
And I hope God gives you the strength to realise
That mummy took a fall and hope that you shall
forgive me
As I still love you all.

Dated: 25th September 1997

Lisa Diallo

Mothers Love

You start your life so helpless,
So frightened and so small
And all the love around you means nothing to you
at all
You took your first breath of air
You opened your tiny eyes
And at that point is when things do change
The most important one our lives

You need to be taken care of, you need a mothers
love
Life so free and gentle, just like a ball of fluff
As each day is done, another day does start
You always touch that special place deep down in
my heart

And now you have reached the age of one
I look back at the work I have done
Sometimes were hard and sometimes were fun
And the only thing now left to say is
I love you
My one and only son.

Dated: 12th April 1992

Journey Into My Life

Dreams Fulfilled

All my life I have wanted a daughter of my own
A little girl, yes a little version of me
My time arrived on the 21st June 1998
A bright and sunny day
That followed by deep blue skies and the heavens
must have opened that day
And sparkled moondust in my eyes

I bore a child, a princess too
She was everything I had asked for, a little girl of
my own
For you gave me everything to live for
And so everyday that I watch you grow
And everyday now we
Know we have each other and there are no words
to explain how I feel
Apart from I am so proud to be your mother

And as each day goes on I love you a little bit more
And I am floating; my feet never seem to touch the
floor
As happiness you brought to my life
As you could possibly bring no other
For my daughter you need to know
I shall forever keep her close and do nothing but
love her

For all my children I have bore
There are no words that can describe
My love, my life, is filled with happiness
And for me that is enough.

Lisa Diallo

All my Life

My daughter is so special, she means everything to me
Without her in my life I could never dream to be
Without her there is no meaning to my life
Without her I am sure I would never of survived

For every smile she gives me and for every laugh I hear
She brings me such happiness and takes away the fear
And everyday as she does grow
Deep in my heart I will always know my love for you can only grow
And here I always will be
Because when I had nothing, you were born
And then at last there was someone that needed me

Throughout her life I will guide her in the best way I know
How to be right
Even though I know that it shall be a struggle and a fight
And when she is older I hope she shall learn
To respect me in every possible way
As that respect I now give her every single day

To my daughter
I love you and everything to you I would give
For you are the reason I still exist
Yes you are the reason why I still live.

Journey Into My Life

Exhausted by Life

All the feeling of exhaustion ready to give in
No point in even trying to get back up
No point in eating and no point in sleeping
Creating dizzy spells and feelings of being sick
These are all that clouds my days
So I wish the lord would call on me and end these
nothing but sad ways

For four children I have bore, all ungrateful and
selfish
And lazy every single one
So please can I have no more
For selfish and inconsiderate they have become
For treated like a cash machine don't even think
they recognise me as mum

For they watch me struggle almost crawling on my
knees
And still they keep just asking
Can I have?
I want never a thank you or a please
Never asking about my needs
Yet miraculously around every payday different
children they become
Even showing slight respect
And when payday is over it all goes back to abuse
and neglect

So angry inside that they can make me feel like this
Thoughts of ending it all, longing to not exist
For my past has only offered me upsets and regrets

Lisa Diallo

Some so severe I shall never be allowed to forget

And so for my children I try the best I can
Hoping for a better life than I did
So why are they so rude and continue to abuse?
Almost feels like they want me to get rid

Rejection is a word that has haunted my life
Some things so young could not have possibly
have been my fault
As far as teenage years go maybe most of that I
brought on myself
Yet no matter what life threw at me I remained
strong
And continued to carry on in the way I knew best

From trying to take my own life
And the drugs, abuse, sex and violent ordeals
The scars from all of these are still fresh and for me
I shall never heal

So I have entered so many phases in my life
Already been married, yes three times a wife
And all I ever longed for was some kind of normality
And from my siblings a little respect
For if only they knew how good it is for them
Never experiencing that familiar word reject

And although on the outside I may appear strong
It's all deceiving so very wrong
As my children have only brought me more hurt
and loss
And so again those feelings of not knowing where I
belong

Journey Into My Life

So now all love is turning into hate
As walking away from them no longer seems so wrong
But do not worry because the old Lisa shall be back before too long

So I have to now decide
Do I put up with this shit?
Or turn my back and walk away? And forever be gone
For there is nothing left for me to do here
Yes everything for me is done

For I know that failure is what everyone expects to see
And as usual all my family just waiting for me to fall
But if no one hears me when I ask for help
Then frustration leading to failure is all that can be gained
For no more of this living hell I can take
There's nothing left but pain

Pro's and con's advantages and disadvantages
I start my list, and they are endless as to whether I stay
As advantages I have listed not one
And the disadvantages to say just go on and on
1001 reasons for me to pack my things up and alone be gone

For I forever have these feelings of rejection
And I am still human
For my mind already has problems of its own
And so now all I can wish for is for everyone to go

Lisa Diallo

Go away and leave me the hell alone
And I shall continue to manage like every time
before with living on my own.

Dated: 19th April 2006

Journey Into My Life

My Heart

A precious person is your gran
And should be loved dearly with all your heart
And so should always be in your thoughts for times
when you're apart

For my gran is an advisor if I needed one
She has been a shelter throughout life's storms
Always offering words of comfort when things did
go wrong
And always gave me that feeling that in her heart I
shall always belong

For gran you are the power and the strength
And you so often freely gave your love
That always went to great lengths
And you showered me with love and affection
And always tried to give me your undivided
attention

For me you shall always be that gran
That made wishes and dreams come true
For you're the one that I admire, respect and adore
As it's you that always gets me through
And everything you mean to me, my heart, my soul,
my inspiration
For you make everything in my life complete.

Dated: January 2004

Lisa Diallo

Thank You

I would like to say Thank You
For all the generous things that you do
As I know that I am lucky to have a gran like you
For sometimes when I am feeling lonely all I have
to do is call
And just knowing you're behind me to catch me if I
should fall

For when God made grandmothers he broke the
mould with you
For somehow you always seemed to manage
Yes you always saw things through
And as I am getting older I would like to think
A role model is you,
For I always seem to admire everything that you do
For you are always helping others no matter what
they do
For you are very special to me
I was just making sure that you knew

So I just wanted to say Thank You
And to let you know you are on my mind
As grandmothers like you are really hard to find
For I only have one grandmother
Is what I now say and together I hope we can make
the most of everyday
For you never know when our precious time will be
taken away.

Dated: 6th May 1998

Journey Into My Life

Thank God I have found you

This year has been so special for me
As my whole life and world was turned around
As even though we have loved and lost
Through it all grandma I have found

And even though I am only little
I still can help a lot
Because there is a part of me that is very special
As I am a reminder of someone that should never
be forgot

But still we would like you to know
That we are always here for you whenever you are
feeling low
For grandma I shall always be around
And that's what I wanted you to know
And for that reason you shall always have a place
to go

So this is a time to be happy
As we welcome in the New Year
But this time we can do it together, and at that point
I shall close my eyes and make a wish
That the rest of our years we shall bring in forever

But for now I shall end this little poem
That has been written especially for you
And there's something else that I wanted you to
know
And that's you are the one
The one that put the sparkle in my eye
As for you I am the memory that shall never die

Lisa Diallo

For it was your son, my dad, that had to say
Goodbye.

Dated: 1st January 2003

Journey Into My Life

Daughters Love

You take it for granted that your mum is always
there
To share your problems and to care
For they try their best to guide you on
On a path they believe to be right
So that this life is a lesser struggle and a fight

But as an individual person you walk your own way
On this journey called life
Always seeming to result in getting stabbed in the
back
With the sharp end of a knife
For you make your own mistakes and never listen
to the truth
And so left always to learn the hard way
I guess its part of our youth

And when the mistakes are made as I did make a
few
I always knew who to turn to
And that person mum, was you
And so now I have a child of my own whom I will
love
In every possible way and always let him know
I'm here for him just like you used to say

So I guess now the time has come
For me to be there for you mum
Although I know that I could never help you in the
ways you have helped me
But I shall try my damned hardest

Lisa Diallo

Because of the love that you always showed to me.

Dated: 28th April 1992

Journey Into My Life

Beauty Within

Never was there a truer saying was that beauty
always comes from within
And since day one a true friend you have been
As your exterior is just a shell
Yes something for everyone to see
But if an angel should look beyond that
Your beauty is more than skin deep

For you carry so much pain deep down inside
Not knowing any way to release
As you have only ever known your feelings to hide
Whether it be through stubbornness
But mainly through so much pride

But I believe in you and I think you should let the
world know
What a truly nice person you are
Believe me your friendship determination and your
dedication
Will take you far

And although right now you may be feeling a little
sad
When it feels like everything you do just turns out
bad
It could be a day a month or even a year
But eventually you shall be glad

Because I believe that things are sent for a reason
So allow fate to take a stern hand
And because of that person you are

Lisa Diallo

I'm sure on your feet you will land.

Dated: 12th April 2003

Journey Into My Life

Someone Special

My special friend how really wonderful you are
You're one in a million; yes you're the best by far
Considerate, grateful, honest
These are but just some of the few things that you
are
For certainly there is no other
That has done for me the things you have done
And still continue to do
There is definitely no other that could have a friend
like you

And so for these reasons is why today
I am sending these words to you
Forever you shall be known as the bestest friend
that I have
And even though arguments and fallouts we shall
occur
They become a thing of the past
For I believe that this friendship is made to last

For no problem or any person
Should be allowed to stand in our way
Of this wonderful friendship
We have worked through and still alive today.

Dated: June 2004

Lisa Diallo

I Feel Your Pain

At this time of worry you are forever in my thoughts
As a friendship like ours is earned through trust
And so therefore is something that can never be bought

And although right now your feelings may be confused
Especially when we are faced with the fact a loved one we may lose
And although I cannot control this
I shall be here in every and anyway
So if you should need me, all you have to do is say

For I know this worry shall result in heartache and pain
And nothing for you shall make sense
And maybe even make you feel like you're going insane
And at that point I want you to remember this one thing
I'm a shoulder to cry on
And love and comfort is what I am offer cause right now that's all I can bring

And for all the reasons above tonight before I lay my head to sleep
I shall pray for your dad and ask the angels to watch over you both
And then to join both you're hearts into one
So you see no matter what then you shall be together

Journey Into My Life

Always shall remain
Even long after he has passed on.

Dated: May 2004

Lisa Diallo

I Am Never Far Away

I know that life is difficult right now
And it makes me sad to see you cry
I would give my soul to the devil for you
I would lie down and die
If only I could take away your pain that you are
feeling
That someone else has caused
But the anger that lies within is stronger
And so violent shall be all it will draw

I often ask myself why people inflict so much pain
upon us
Especially when the ones closest to our hearts
Seems they are never satisfied with stabbing you in
the back
They then go on to proceed in going and tearing
you apart

And although I know did contribute
As argue over me you did do
But when all else fails I will be the one
That is still there to help you pull through

So no matter which way you choose to play your
cards
Either way it is going to be hard
As this shall be another one of life's little tests
And all you have to remember is to look after
number one
And leave everyone else to rest

Journey Into My Life

And at these times one thing I want you to
remember
Always that is no matter what you go through
I shall not be very far, my love to you shall always
find

And the one thing that I ask in return from you
Is not to let this hurt carry on
For if it continues then just pack his bags and let
him be gone

I feel your anger when you hurt
And I feel sad when I see you cry
But we both know deep down that the truth lies not
very far behind
So let go now do not continue
To live this lie
Funny now how I find myself saying certain things
to you
That you once said to me
And as usual did ignore
And now all seems clear, now I understand
That you just did not want me to hurt anymore

For I know in the past we have been enemies
And so time apart we did have
Yet even still my heart still feels
And my eyes still reveal all when I am sad
And so they say that blood is thicker than water
That you keep dangling on a thread

So if anything else does occur
And you find that it leaves you feeling sad
If life makes you angry and forever feeling bad

Lisa Diallo

Just call on me as I shall always be near
As my love is unconditional
And for you shall always remain clear
Without it you shall never have to fear
For a few chosen words is what you shall hear

For I love you and I care
And I want these words to remain in your head
And so for the times when you shall be feeling low
You can remember these words that to you I once
said.

Dated: 7th November 2002

Journey Into My Life

Chapter 3

1. Made to Last
2. Living Without You
3. Final Thoughts
4. As Time Goes By
5. In love with I fell
6. Judgement Day
7. Nothing changes just sit and wait
8. Because I are
9. Sorry
10. Where did the love go
11. Grateful
12. Stubborn Pride
13. Say Goodbye
14. Calm before the storm
15. One Way Track
16. You can't play a player
17. Floating
18. Worlds Apart
19. Heart full of love
20. Mind Games
21. Soul Mate
22. I do
23. Emptiness
24. Another year over
25. A lesson learnt
26. Ready to give in
27. Right Here
28. What If…
29. Someone out there
30. Distance apart grows fonder the heart
31. Breathe Again

Journey Into My Life

Made to Last

I have had some time
To sort things out in my head
And feelings for you is what I did find
But then the problems arise due to distance and our lack of time
For I still remember when my eyes met yours
They opened every closing door
And have answered every question that I have asked
So many times before

But now my heart and mind is filled with only love for you
But deep down only uncertainties and doubts
Leaves only thoughts of not knowing what to do
I know that I love you for that I cannot change
So why are so many obstacles being put in our way?
For we are both two grown adults with minds of our own
And even though we love each other
Then answer me why are we both still so alone?

For we are living two separate lives
Yet sharing both our hearts
For I hold one half and you have the other part
But still in my heart and thoughts
One day we can be together and forever I shall wish us to stay
So then let's make the most of every waking day

Lisa Diallo

Now certain things have happened
That only led me to believe it was never meant to be
Too much distance between us
Love is blind
Or was it that I just refused to see

One thing I wanted to say, there are no regrets not even one
It was that all the hurt and sadness started to overpower all the fun
But still no matter where life does lead us no matter where we go
I shall always love you, and so for now that is all you need to know.

Dated: 29th May 1992

Journey Into My Life

Living Without You

When you are away life gets harder everyday
Without your arms to gently comfort me or your lips
to gently kiss me
I'm left wondering if you miss these things too
Everyday I long to hold you
Obey yet control you
Forever hold on tight
Take away the darkness and brighten up the nights

Without you the sun never seems to shine
The brightness of the sun causing me to become
blind
But never doubting at any point that you are solely
mine
I cannot imagine this life without you
So all the sad things we should not dwell
And all the feelings of truth to each other we should
tell

For one day I dream that we shall be together
And then the nights will no longer be cold
As when you embrace me the security of your arms
in my memory
I shall forever hold

And as everyday then that shall pass us by
I dream at the end of our days we shall remember
only the love that we felt
And not of the sorrows it sometimes dealt
As from the day we met you my heart did melt.

Dated: February 1996

Lisa Diallo

Final Thoughts

I feel our relationship is not working out
For always in my mind I recognise the deceit
Leaving nothing but doubts
And so many things have happened that we can
never change
Only tears and bad memories of us is now what
remains

I know I am not perfect
But not many people are
But too much water has gone under the bridge
I think this time we have pushed our luck too far
For it seems nothing is left between us
Yes our bridges have already been burnt down
As I feel like any love you held for me is nowhere to
be found

I guess that time just grew between us
Separating our two hearts
As all the hurt and sorrow just now seems like a
farce
For we have tried so many times before to make
this relationship work
But our pasts we can never forget
For somehow and sometime it always seems to
lurk

For our memory does not allow us to forget all
The past hurt upset and anger
That caused us to break so many times before

Journey Into My Life

And for this is a reality check that cannot be ignored
Although last night we spent together
Everything was different as just lust is all I did see
For what we made was like nothing like the love making we had before
And I know now that can never be

But ten out of ten for effort yes I believe we really did try
Effort was definitely done
But this time around baby, its game set and match
Because this time nobody won.

Dated: 6th November 1999

Lisa Diallo

As Time Goes By

I remember the day we were married
Those sacred words 'I do'
In sickness and in health, in poverty and wealth
But what did they mean to you?
Although you tried your hardest
Our marriage still persisted to fail
I guess for me I was just too young as I forever
wanted to bail

Four years later reunited we became
Some people did say we were being foolish
Everyone thought we were going insane
But we were just trying to capture all that love that
we never found
And at the point I was pleased that you were
around

But somewhere on our journey we lost ourselves
In time I thought everything was rosy
And that we were doing just fine
But then I found that your heart did wander as I
believe now
That it lay with someone else
I guess you could say that this is my payback
For that raw deal that to you I once dealt

I tried to be honest and to give you all that I had left
to give to you
I guess I thought that somehow together we could
revive that old flame
That we once knew

Journey Into My Life

But things were dead and buried
We were finally through.

Dated: 7th July 2001

Lisa Diallo

In Love With You I Fell

In married life there are always ups and downs
As no two people are the same
As sometimes we believe that we are always right
Or is it just that we are too ashamed to accept the blame

Yet even so joined together as one
For now is the time for both of us to learn about each other
Some believe a lifetime it can take
But instead of learning about each others faults
Be impulsive and live for one another

Why is it that people say we should wait a year or two?
Until we pledge our vows
Cause there's one thing this life has taught me
Feeling are what your heart controls
And even though there shall be rows
So what if it is ten years or even ten day's time
Cannot control if you will love more or less
But once you have had that feeling inside
It will be then that you know how it feels to experience the best

For only a short while me and my husband have been joined
'Together'
And still each other we shall never fully know
But as long as we do this together we can enjoys the highs

Journey Into My Life

And forever survive the lows

I never did believe in love at first sight
Until my husband Mamadou
For it was the soft look in his eyes, his gentle touch
I felt I could read his mind
Then before I was aware in love with him I fell
So quickly yet so deep
Feelings that I was no longer in control
And that my heart on me was ready to cheat

There was no time to hold back
No realisation of what was going on all around
For the first sign of reality was when I was stood
taking my vows
And I turned to look in his eyes
And it was then that I knew a husband for life I had
found

And even though sometimes we shall make each
other angry
Causing us to react in unusual ways
I want you to know that I would never turn back the
clock
For it's with you that I wish to spend the rest of my
days

As someone did say
Live for today and not for tomorrow
Be grateful for the nights and appreciate all days
spent together
Replenish all sorrows, enjoy each moment that we
share
For true love is for keeps

Lisa Diallo

It's not something that you can borrow

For even though I do not know
Where this short journey in life shall end
Whether we are parted or remain together
For me there shall never be another
As I am planning on loving you forever

So if I should die tomorrow
My soul can lay to rest
As God to me was good
As he brought me Mamadou Diallo
As this time he sent me the best
And for every problem that we dealt with
And every obstacle that may stand in our way
If our love for each other is stable and strong
Then nothing we shall do shall go wrong

So with these words I note a special date
February 21st 2004
And many more years we shall celebrate this as
one
For I love you with all my heart
I guess this time I finally won
So love honour and obey
And also the words I do
In my heart you shall always remain.

Dated: March 2002

Journey Into My Life

Judgement Day

So here comes the tester
Here comes the big day
As I shall not know if you are coming home
Or if they decide to lock you away
The day seemed to last forever, every noise and
every sound
I would pause, stop and listen just in case your
voice I could hear
As every thought I now have is turning into fear

Remembering our last kiss
And remembering our parting words
And wondering how soon it would be before I would
hear them again
For time has no essence every second seemed to
drag
And every minute feels like hours
I think I am slowly going insane

Reminiscing of the times when I have looked in
your eyes
And everything I did see
Especially all the love you held for me
And then at that point togetherness was what I
wanted you and me to be
For you made me feel like no other person has
before
You gave me the space, to find myself
And my feelings to explore

Lisa Diallo

Just one example when I was blind you helped me to see
When I lost my way it was you who cleared the path ahead for me
And for the times when I was laying frail on the floor
Then you picked me up and loved me some more

And as all these thoughts questioned my mind
Feeling for you I am starting to find
But yet still not knowing if we should have a future together
Whether we carry out our promise to remain
With each other forever

Then as I stare from my daze of thoughts of me and you
I thought that I saw your face
Blocked by the bright sunshine shining through
And as I rubbed my eyes for now to see clear
I thanked the lord above that he had brought you back here

And for all this I was thankful
And content that night as I lay my head to sleep
For I know together safe is what the lord will keep
So I prayed that night that we should never be apart
The truth now being I do not think I could take another broken heart.

Dated: 10th October 2003

Journey Into My Life

Nothing changes just sit and wait

My life seems always the same, no one there to turn to
Yet again guess I am the one that shall take the blame
In a relationship I am supposed to be
So then I am left asking myself
Why is he not here with me?

Hour after hour left to just sit and wait
And time is slowly ticking away
And yet again it's getting rather late
But eventually he will show
Expecting everything to be fine, but feelings are getting hurt
But why are they always mine?

Always thinking where he is and questioning myself
About what he is doing?
How many more times must I sit and wait
How many times do I sit and debate about where he goes and what he does
The answer seems simple
To end this relationship, I only wish I could

But every time I try to end this waiting and hurt
I feel as though my heart is burnt
But nothing changes and here I sit still
There is no one that gives a shit
I wish I could only think of myself and never give a care
This torment that pulls out my heart

Lisa Diallo

I guess I shall never know.

Dated: August 1998

Journey Into My Life

Because I care

I know that you think I nag too much
But the reason for this is you see
It's because I love you and you mean so much too me
To ignore things would be easier
Yes to pretend that there is nothing wrong
But as we both definitely know
That problem will be back before too long

I cannot adopt this attitude and maybe one day shall see why
For every given moment is there for me and you to try
And then someday in the future it may even be when I am gone
You will sit and think of me
Then realise why I soften kept nagging on

Although between us driving a distance
It's now obvious to see and is sure only to bring pain
But maybe if we could get through together
We shall see the bright sunshine then do away with the drizzle of rain

I often sit and think of you
Well actually a lot, trying not to push my luck
And remembering not to lose the plot
But still I pray things between us shall get better
And all the joys will overcome the power of the pain
Brought by loving you

Lisa Diallo

For it shall never feel like a bind
But for both of us be a gain.

Dated: 4th May 2004

Journey Into My Life

Sorry

For all the pain I have caused you
For all the hurt you have felt
For all the tears that you shed
And all the sorrows that I have dealt

I would like to say sorry…

For all the times I did not hold you
For all the times I did not say I love you
For all the wrong that I did
And for all the wrongs I still do

I would like to say sorry…

I know how much I need you
And I know how much I want you
So I guess sorry is not the word I need
And I shall try a little bit harder
Because I want us to be together
Because baby it's on your love that I feed.

So I would like to say I love you.

Dated: June 1999

Lisa Diallo

Where did the love go?

How did we ever get to this?
I remember how it all started out, with one small gentle kiss
And so from all the love and warmth around us
Yet now to cold lonely nights
I ask myself where did the love go?
At which point did it turn to arguments and fights

For every time that communication did break down
For 2 or 3 days sometimes more
I find that I am asking myself what happened to that man I married?
The one I used to love and adore

With you I felt every emotion possible
And I think I shed every tear that my eyes allowed me to cry
As I feel that we are slowly drifting apart
So much that you are barely in sight
And so your love for me I assume is about ready to die

For each time we did not speak
And just ignored the situation at hand
It makes me feel like a floating kite just waiting for the wind
To stop causing me to crash land
And the thing that I fear most of all is that each time it is getting easier
I no longer feel pain when you walk out that door

Journey Into My Life

I live everyday with the fear of uncertainty
Of that one day it shall all be gone
All the love trapped inside of me and is screaming
to get out
But only you hold the key and when you release
You will then see what you mean to me

But still if there is any doubt in your mind about our
future together
Then all I ask is for you to be honest and just tell it
as it is
And then either way I want you to know that forever
I shall love you
As you stole a piece of my heart
And that shall never change as I promised to death
do us part.

Dated: September 2004

Lisa Diallo

Grateful

I needed you to know that I am grateful
For all the things that you do
Although I often shout and scream it's not
necessarily down to you
Sometimes I get so low there never seems to be
any signs
It feels like sometimes we are just living a lie

I know in the past I have not made your life easy
And I guess you cannot say I still don't
But that does not mean it is beyond me
It doesn't mean that I won't
I guess we never had a chance to make things
easy
But one day I am sure we will get there
As this life has dealt us a lot of raw deals
I am sure by now it is about time life treated us both
fair

Although joined together like man and wife
We could never be
I will always have love and respect for you
As in the meantime I have known you, you have
always given to me
These few words I sent to you probably do not
make a lot of sense
But can answer what in life does

For as long as we look after each other
And most of all the kids
Then who cares what anyone else has to say

Journey Into My Life

Just tell them to put a lid on it
What I am trying to say is thank you
For giving me another chance to be with my kids
again
And the same to turn my life around
For without these chances you gave me I would
have ended up six foot underground.

Dated: 3rd June 2001

Lisa Diallo

Stubborn Pride

Forever letting your stubborn pride get in the way
Always allowed it to make others pay
And for awhile I guess I did
But then you forgot to end the game and so eventually
It was me that was pleased to of got rid

Pride with yourself is always a good thing
Putting pride before others can only be a sin
As bringing with it a sense of power way beyond compare
Taking over you, never noticing that you was not being fair

After you walked away
Some kind of control freak must have entered your soul
As every decision to be made you felt that had to be yours
And every part of me you must own
Looking for a compromise but only your way
I do as you say or you will stay away
Did you ever limit?
On how many times I had to suffer, how many times did you want me to pay?

Forever deceit and lies is what came
And so for me brought only tears and pain
Forever wondering what it was that you wanted to achieve

Journey Into My Life

I believe only to break my heart then to continue
tearing it apart
And even that was not enough
I was willing to do anything you wanted
Was even happy for you to remain in control
Because I was so in love with you
But you continued the heartache and then
continued to dish up more

I know I have been heartless in my past
And so I guess karma came back around on this
player
But never once did my heart stray
Just forever looking for ways to make me love you
again
I would have moved mountains and even walked
the wire
Even as extreme as walking on fire
Just for you to love me again

But it was at that point that I got to wondering
Yes to wondering how someone could walk away
from someone so easily
That they are supposed to love
Not even giving any chances or pulling things back
together
So please excuse my bluntness baby
But when I married you I vowed before friends and
family
That I would love you forever

Yes forever together
Destined, we were meant to be
So wrapped up in you that I was too blind to see

Lisa Diallo

I don't think you had any love for me
Well not real love
Not like it is supposed to be
Always talking of your wedding ring leaves me with
only one question
'Why did you marry me?'
Why not do the kindest of things and let me remain
free

As I have often spoke about before
You ended my childhood fairy dream
And you changed all the rules for I was supposed
to live happily ever after
With you by my side
Now I have nothing left to believe in
Because you have taken it all away
And just like the fairytale you have faded out
With the night of day

Maybe now you have caused me suffering and pain
Please tell me Mamadou
What was your gain?

Dated: 17th July 2005

Journey Into My Life

Say Goodbye

In a world where nothing stays the same
But this time I am not about to take the blame
For all the pain you caused me, for all the hurt you
dealt
You never once looked back to ask how I really felt

The hurt in my eyes became too easy to see
So advantage you then took and set out to hurt me
As I dropped my defences and began to show you
my love
But yet even though this was hard for me to do
You still persisted on destroying me and you

Physically you hurt me but it was mentally that you
left scars
So yet again my defences come up
And once again I learnt how to be hard
Now my barriers are solid never brought down
Silent now is my love for you, never to make
another sound

For in love with you so deep I fell
Sometimes it felt like heaven
But eventually you created a living hell
But for all the love that I still feel forever now I shall
never reveal
For I dreamed one day to marry, yes be your wife
But you became determined to only destroy two
people's lives.

Dated: 22nd August 2001

Lisa Diallo

Calm before the Storm

Everything now feels perfect
Seems like everything is finally going our way
For more in love with you I fall every single day
But still in the back in my mind something niggles
Wondering when someone shall take it away

As from past experiences I have come to learn that somehow
This is the calm before the storm
Like the peaceful nights, followed the by the chaos of the dawn
For never have I known for things to feel so right
I have never felt happy as I do right now
For it is the lord above that made this happen so on my bended knees
I bow

In just a matter of days you have turned my life around
From sadness and all the everyday problems
And my head full of self doubts for you have now become everything
I have dreamed of and more
Yet still a little hesitant to believe
Praying never again to see you walk out that door

Finding it hard to believe how you are making me feel
For so much love and contentment is now what you deal
Yes a feeling that of somewhere I belong

Journey Into My Life

The feeling of trust that I am building in you
But still at the back of my mind
Wondering when will be the next time that you say
we are through

But I hope all the words that you say are coming
from deep down in your heart
Feeling you have kept locked up inside
Protecting yourself from any hurt from the start
But I want you to know that every moment we
share
That we confess how we feel
It's those words that help me survive everyday
Because when all else fails and everything goes
wrong
I know that you are coming home to me
For in my heart is where you belong

I promise you know that I shall never abuse your
love
Or use your feelings to play around
Because now I believe true love is what I have
found
So let's set our aims high now
For to aim in only each other to love
For now I believe that being with you shall for me
always be enough.

Dated: 9th August 2004

One Way Track

Looking and searching but yet never to find
The questions all there, but still no answers come
to mind
I know what I want but somehow I fear
These feelings I have will one day disappear

So my answer to this is just to hold back
I feel like a train on a one way track
Never turning any corners, never trying a new route
My life's one long journey
Of which I am not sure as to whether I can see it
through

When I try to explain how I feel
I get so angry deep inside, and I hate everything
about me
But still these thoughts I try to deny
For that better person inside I still long to find
I find it hard to believe that anyone could love me,
just for being me
I often refuse to believe it as I believe there is a
price tag that goes with it
I am always looking to see

I suppose deep down I want to be a better person
And change the hurt that is within me
As I know deep down inside my inner self
A better person I know I shall see

I know I am capable of giving my love
But I have problems of it being returned

Journey Into My Life

And for this it has caused me heartache all
throughout my life
For my feelings I always seem to fight

I guess I need to learn how to love and not to be
frightened
To be loved back
I guess now I need to change my destination
And get off that one way track, for this life is no
game that we play
It's not fiction for this life is a real fact.

Dated: 21st November 2002

Lisa Diallo

You can't play a player

Very good now
You're a player, go ahead and talk your talk
But one thing you need to ask yourself
Is can you walk the walk?
Ok so now you start to raise your voice so that
everyone can hear
What you think you're a player?
And what? Am I supposed to fear you?
So what is it baby do you think I am scared that
maybe
You will say we're through
Oh baby oh baby
If only you knew

So next time when you wish to chat about your next
catch
Please don't mind me, but please remember to
close the door on the way out
Cause if you want to play then I cannot get down
with you anymore
So I will just take myself up to the club
The same place that I found you
Then I will just trade you in for someone spanking
new

And I guess now you think you are clever
Thinking that me and you have played
Thinking you caught me out cause I don't know you
strayed
Well I am sorry to say I got bad news for you
Cause you have not played this player

Journey Into My Life

For when you got on your knees to praise I was on mine too
Yes I was the one that was playing long before you even knew

So look who's laughing now babe
I think maybe this one is for me
For when I was calling out someone else's name
You was too blind to see
So you can keep your word love and I shall accept
That you're meaning of marriage is another word for a joke
As all those feelings I once held for you meant nothing now to me
And from now on I shall always be one step ahead
And every time I will rise above you as if I am guilty of doing wrong
Then that was only to love you
But even that was not enough for the shit you put me through.

Dated: 14th September 2004

Floating

I am 29 years of age and yet I am still floating
Somewhere in between lives wondering where I will
end up
I still do not know where to go; I crave for someone
to hold
Yet my feelings I still find hard to show

Although I am grateful, as I have four children
Who I am proud of in every single way
They make my life worth living, they brighten up
every day
And a few simple words like I love you mummy is
all they have to say

People say never judge a book by its cover
And in my case it's true, I smile I laugh
Even crack a joke or two but nobody knows what's
inside
If only they knew

I hurt like everyone else, I cry like all humans do
I guess some people would say that I am crazy
But the saddest thing is that it is the truth
Disappointed people have been by my actions
And also by what I say
But if they knew what I am going through
They would wonder how I get by some days
Some days I don't want to wake up, my only wish is
to die

Just once in awhile I long for those words

Journey Into My Life

That lets you know that someone cares
I need someone beside me through the obstacles
and the temptations and dares
Just to know I w ill survive and see my children
grow
At least to the point when I am grey and old

In my life I have not achieved alot but I do not really
care
As I have experienced every way of life, the love
the hurt
And learned how people can be unfair
But one thing I can be proud of is the children I
have bore
Because when this life offers me nothing
I can ignore hateful words around me
The violence and the hate stay behind my doors

So all I ask out of this joke called life
Is that when my children are older and go their
separate ways
That they remember the good times that we spent
with the fun filled days

Because without memories we cannot survive
And without dreams it seems pointless carrying on
But with the memories we capture
No one can take them away
Yes over the years the things we have done
No one can take them away, no one has a say

So to my children for when you are older
If at any point this poem you should see
Keep all your memories and thoughts together

Lisa Diallo

And I pray that you think of me.

Dated: 30th November 2001

Journey Into My Life

Worlds Apart

Breakdown of communication
I was always saying it would get worse
As I always knew that deep down it would break us
What I did not realise is that I would be the one to give in first
Yes the first to give in as throughout became a tug of war
But eventually no battles did either of us win

And even though without you it's destined that I would hurt so deep down
The scars would be left to remain
Although on the outside will show different you will find
But really it's all just blown my mind

For too many times have I opened my heart to you
And let my thoughts and feelings out and instead of taking them down
You walked over them leaving me with only hurt anger and doubts

But I must admit I never really knew
What being in love was like until that day I met you
As somehow unaware your love crept in
And my heart you managed to get in
Still to this day I cannot explain why or how these feelings I had
All that I know for certain is that
Out of me you brought out every emotion
Happiness love and tears

Lisa Diallo

But then eventually you turned it all bad

So even though we fell to pieces I refuse to carry the blame
For I lost count of the many times that I backed down
Just to end the mind games
Yet confrontation was never your strong point as you would rather ignore
In the hope that it would go away
But like I said too many times before
It escalates and then returns in a bigger way

And every time ignorance you did deal
A piece of my heart you gave back
And for that I started to again become strong and then for me
Everything suddenly became clear
That from the beginning everything about me and you was wrong
And so at that point I knew together we did not belong

But again on a serious note I did not regret
A single thing for all was put there for us to learn
And not all of it was doom and gloom
But for all the bad times the end was inevitable
Just feels like it came too soon

But still I wish you well
Wherever or whatever you choose to do
But I hope that you have learnt one thing from these experiences and mistakes
And pray that this life you shall get through.

Journey Into My Life

Heart full of Love

This morning when I woke up I did not know
What for me was in store, another day I used to say
another closing door
Yet little did I know today that my door would open
wide
And my heart would come aglow
Because now I know that in you
I have found a love that keeps me a flow

I look in your eyes, they reveal all the warmth
The love you have for me, and it was at that point
I realised that we were meant to be
When you enter the room my heart filled with only
love for you
As you have become the reason that now gets me
through

I do not want to have to live without you; I hope I
never have to
But only time will tell and cast a spell
And forever keep our love alive

All we have to remember is to stick close together
and to follow our dreams
Even when we feel like we are falling apart at the
seams
For if one day the knot we should tie and that I shall
become your wife
For you to me are everything, yes baby I made you
my life.

Dated: December 2003

Mind Games

Why is it that still as adults we insist on playing mind games?
It just seems to me that as we get older
The rules become a little more advanced
For they offer no mercies and there is nothing left for a second chance

To get into someone's head and have the power to make them believe
That what you're saying is true
Such a wonderful blessed gift
Yet abused by everyone, especially me and you

But to me it only brings one reminder
A saying I have so often heard
For we are only going around in circles
Losing all love and ability to care, some people are weak and some are strong
I am not talking about physically but also mentally
As we all need somewhere to belong

Mental stimulation and the power to control someone's mind
I assume that it was never created for us to use for hate
And maybe was given for a much better use
Yet this world is filled with so much anger and betrayal
Leaves us mentally weak and physically frail

So I sit here today to ask myself

Journey Into My Life

Why so much pleasure is found in controlling
someone's mind
What are these people seeking?
I know not why they are hoping to find

All the weak minded people are played on the most
And sometimes even driven to take their own lives
Where as the strong minded somehow manage to
survive this life

I believe that it is what's in your heart and how
much you can trust yourself
Stubbornness and selfishness sometimes can
become your strength
To believe in yourself body and mind
I think maybe is the answer I have been looking to
find.

Dated: 21st April

Lisa Diallo

Soul Mate

You entered my life so swiftly
Instantly we did bond
As something strange did happen that day
As straight away of you I became fond
Conversation was flowing like we had known each
other for years
There was no uncomfortable silences, no stress
And of each other we held no fears

As time went by, we did meet again
For longer than the last and still again I felt like I
knew you
Like someone from my past
And before I had time to realise
I found myself missing you every day
Unfortunately our time together was cut short as
you lived so far away

As you was leaving to go back home
A lump appeared in my throat
And then my stomach turned when you reached for
your coat
And so was feeling really silly as we had not known
each other long
Left all thoughts inside my head
Which is where I thought best belonged

Now time alone I find myself
Yet every time my mind drifted to you
Sometimes leaving me feel a little sad
And also feeling blue

Journey Into My Life

And finally when things got me down and I did not
feel I could not go on
My instant reaction was to call you
Yes you became my number one

Then I decided it only fair to let you know
As to relieve your mind of any doubts
So I decided to break it down baby
And said to you let's all go out
Yes let these feelings go deep inside each others
hearts
And take these chances and risks
As you are my number one
Yes baby it's you that is on the top of my list

So I decided not to be scared and show my feelings
to you
That my past so often did abuse
So I followed my hearts intuition and decided that
you're the one
The person I did not want to lose

So these words are a reminder
Of when we first met
That we can look back on it in years to come
And so now we are joined together
True love for me and for you is finally done
This time we won.

Dated: 19th November 2004

Lisa Diallo

I Do

Those binding words that we spoke together
Were declarations of our love to each other
For the rings that we exchanged
Were the tokens of the legal binding of two hearts
A promise to each other that we shall never part

As we both promised to remain supportive of each
other
And give the freedom to be totally honest with each
other
We shall laugh and cry together
And together strive to achieve all our goals by
setting our aims high
And it is then that this world should offer us no
more goodbyes

But most important to love and cherish, honour and
obey
In sickness and in health, through poverty stricken
times
Yet also through all the wealth
And most of all to remain honest to me and
importantly to yourself

These words shall now become our memories
Of the vows we pledge to each other
When in matrimony we were joined together
When to all those vows we did say, and the
exchanging of rings
Finalises our commitment that our future together
shall bring.

Journey Into My Life

Emptiness

Empty inside, going nowhere
All alone yet still these feelings of wanting to hide
But hide from what I question myself
Maybe it's of the feelings I have inside

Wanting to call someone or even better to have someone here
Even if only to protect me of my own inner fears
But yet again another failing side of my life
Relationships are not for me, for three times already been a wife

For a good man I can never seem to find
For when I do I throw it all away
Always assuming that eventually they shall stray
So I guess I am now made to pay like this
For nothing lasts forever and happiness for me is on a very short list

So I remain alone sat wondering if anyone I shall even find
And have a relationship, one of a lasting kind
Dreaming of what life's supposed to be like
Remembering fairytales of old
The kind that you could never buy and could never be sold

Led all those years to believe that's how life really is
How that fairytale dream I had I now do miss
Where did things go so very wrong?

Lisa Diallo

And how from that did I get to this?

For I do not remember the princess being lonely or
even feeling this sad
For happily ever after is what they had
For this was only the one thing that I had left to
believe in
But now reality shows me how I have nothing
And like that old fairytale dream everything
becomes a reality
And just like everything else in my life, it's been and
gone now.

Dated: 9th February 2006

Journey Into My Life

Another Year Over

Well another year is over, and so another one does start
Supposedly joy and celebrations and affairs of the heart
People joining together, no time for fighting or even being torn apart

So I guess then it's just me again!
The one that's sat all alone
My only contact with the outside world is texting me on my phone
Although a few surprises were waiting in store
No knocks on the front door
Just an ex-husband on the telephone

Yes surprise surprise
Out of the woodwork he did crawl
Still cannot believe that he wants to spend his New Years Eve with me
Or is he just building me up for another fall
Because now he can see yet again I am standing tall
Yes rose above it all

While present loved ones yet again choose to play games
Funny how at times like these, their minds choose to stray
Well 2005 I left it all alone and I brought 2006 in alone too
So I guess the proof's in the pudding here

Lisa Diallo

It's just the single for me
Oh what again?!

But still I shall not let things get me down, but just
the same
As the last I shall make my resolutions knowing
damn well
Like everything else, they're not bound to last.

Dated: 1st January 2006

Journey Into My Life

A Lesson Learnt

A lesson in life's situations taken for granted you
would always care
For a chance on your feelings I took to dare
Never appreciated just what I had and never
realised how happy you made me
Forever I only seemed to make you mad

But then life leads us into situations where reality
turns around
Kicks us from behind
But when you really need somebody, you turn
around
But no one you can find

For now I admit that I so often took your love for
granted
Assumptions led me to believe that you would
always be there
And no matter what happened I always believed
you would care
If only I could have realised that your heart I did
care

So I guess I am writing these few words to you
With all the apologies I could send
And even though it can never be enough I hope
someday that you could forgive me
And then forever remain friends
And then all those bridges that I burnt down
Hopefully I shall fully mend

Lisa Diallo

For a hard and harsh lesson I have learnt
I know in my heart for me was severe
For now I live with my feelings of emptiness along
with my dread of fear
Never to feel the warmth of true and unconditional
love again
Something that you used to so freely give
For the tender kiss and gentle touch all these things
are now
Is what is left for me to reminisce

If I had known how much I was hurting you
I would have never of you took for granted and
would have been grateful
And appreciative of each loving word that to me
you spoke
Instead I know that I abused your trust and so often
did provoke
But now what went around just came around
I fear I'm living in hell and for all the times I abused
your love
Is all I now have to sit and dwell?

Dated: 25th March 2004

Journey Into My Life

Ready to give in

Constant pains everyday
Inside my head feels like I am going insane
For several months in silence I have now suffered
The continuous pains in my head
My teeth, my feet, everyday something breaks
down and no solutions offered
Especially no relief

Just one whole day to be free of all pain
For this is the only one thing that I have now left to
gain
For it's my only wish right now as I am forever
unhappy
Forever feeling sad, as my internal system seems
all to be turning bad
Although I admit it is my own entire fault
As self neglect over the years of my body inside
and out
Ready to give in feels like I am a prisoner still
waiting to get out

For over the years I have driven myself into the
ground
For my state of mind there's only bits left to find
Now all thoughts fill my head with negative
thoughts
But today myself I have taught, even though I kneel
to pray
I wish my lord oh my life please take today

For inside I am dying and outside I'm left crying

Lisa Diallo

For no medication now seems to work
Drastic measures as I pop another pill already
knowing the quantity I have taken
It's going to make me ill
Still I try to laugh never knowing pain like this
before
Dragging myself along the floor, already climbed up
every wall
Begging anyone please make it stop, I cannot take
much more.

Dated: 20th September 2004

Journey Into My Life

Right Here...

Feelings of excitement mixed with feelings of fear
Still finding it hard to believe your really here
Feels like all my dreams have now come true
And it's all because of you

When we did part from our lives together
Without you I thought I would be forever
Always looking for ways to win back your heart
But all I succeeded to do was drive us further apart

So when you decided to move towns
Just try to imagine how many days I felt down
For I thought I would never see you again
As your wife or a lover or even a friend
And I promised myself that I would get through with
my broken heart
As it was then that I realised forever we would be
apart

But today you are here right in front of my very
eyes
Promising that these tears of joy I would not cry
Hearing those words that for me you still feel a little
And agreeing to try again
Feels like I have just found that long lost lover and
friend.

Dated: 29th January 2006

What if…

One minute you are here but only in body not in mind
And I know your heart and soul left long ago
All I wish that I had known at what point you were breaking
If only you had told me before
That you were ready to give in that you were ready to let go

And for that now all that I am left with is questions
And wondering if you ever loved me at all
Questioning did you love me at the start
Or was it all a false pretence
Or was there really a place for me in your heart

It was once said that love is very close to lust
And therefore becomes hard to define the truth between the two
Which yet again gets me to wondering if you knew yourself?
As you walked away easily and said we were finally through

Or what if you did really love me?
Somewhere down deep in your heart yet somehow we drifted apart
And just went through the motions not even knowing ourselves
Maybe you felt pressured into the marriage
Maybe you would have preferred me as a friend
But baby

Journey Into My Life

If so the wrong signals you did send

And I guess now I could sit for hours, days, even weeks
Just asking myself,
'What if?'
Just to then find that reality kicks you from behind
Then all that's left is just memories of me and you to miss

Yet still funny how life turns out
As we drifted apart as swiftly as we were brought together
Never taking the time to discover anything about each other
No time to find or learn as friends or lovers

I figured out we tried to run before we could walk
We was singing out loud before we could even talk
The other option being the grim reality
Saying maybe we were never meant for each other
Yet still from the start I have never wanted to be with another
I believed we were meant to be

Together was like fire fighting fire
Always doubting each other made us no longer strong
Just tired of the fighting with each other
Resulting in us making nothing but good liars

But at that point, where we started lying to ourselves
We only brought hatred and pain

Lisa Diallo

The end result was that enemies we became
When really instead of dividing ourselves we should
have made each other feel
Make us feel equally the same

And yet all the assumptions and all the maybes
Are just thoughts we hold in our mind
But that is when the reality and the truth become
unbearable to define
Yet still despite the uncertainties of us
And also the insecurities of myself, the arguments,
the fears, worries and doubts
And through all the tears and emotions there was
one thing
Of which I was always sure and throughout always
remained
My mind was playing the game but my heart was
starting to ache

For the kisses I missed and the smallest things you
used to say
Although not spoken often
As that would change the rules of the game
It was then I thought I could take on the world
You made me believe I was like a movie star
That had just reached their fame

Yet now in a matter of days
My self confidence, my smile, my heart, a piece of
me you did take
And for the first time in my life
I found out what it was like to have my heart to
break
But one thing you should know

Journey Into My Life

Whatever you're reasoning for marrying me
I can honestly say that mine were true
Never once was anything false or faked
For I was a hundred per cent dedicated to you.

Dated: 3rd April 2004

Someone Out There

To have so much yet so little is how I always feel
Somewhere out there I know this life has to be
ready to offer me a fair deal
Yet still there is something that is missing
I keep searching but never can find
But I have my four children so to a certain extent
life is treating me kind

Relationships, they always come second
But with this I know not what to do
There is always that someone special
There is always me and you
Some people would say I have everything, but if
that as true
Then why does my heart feel so sad?
Yes I have my children whom I love in everyway
So why do I feel I am just ticking away the days?

It feels like a life long calendar and each day it gets
ticked away
But to myself I ask
What shall my aim be?
When will I reach the final day?
As when I find a goal in life I feel then my life will be
complete
For everyday is an uphill battle
Yet all I seem to claim is defeat

Some people may say I want too much out of this
life
Then show me someone who doesn't

Journey Into My Life

Oh yes I've had the career, the wife and four times I
am a mother
Yet still to this day I feel like there is more waiting
ahead
That I know I can achieve
I think they call it self satisfaction, so for me
I guess my aim in life is in myself I have to believe.

Dated: 7th February 2002

Lisa Diallo

Distance apart grow fonder the heart

Sat alone with words going through my head
At 2.30am knowing I really should be tucked up in
my bed
But every minute of the day thoughts of you will not
go away
Remembering all those things we said

Sat all alone just thinking of you wondering if you
are missing me too
As the distance between us seems so very far
Longing to hold you, knowing that I can't brings me
Only sadness to my heart

Yet when I sit and analyse
I know I should be grateful for what I have got
As it was only a few months ago I thought I had lost
the lot
So now I am counting the days till I see you again
And I shall hold onto tighter than ever before
For it is then that I know the distance can offer so
much more

For it was once said that distance makes the heart
grow fonder
And so on that statement I now do ponder
And for the first time I saw the sense of it all
Things I never really could understand before
For every time we were apart I miss you from the
bottom of my heart
Yes I miss you that little bit more

Journey Into My Life

Yet when we were again joined together it's then that I am
Reminded that I shall love you forever.

Dated: 16th February 2006

Breathe Again

For every breath I take, I take it for you
Every dream I dream is for my love for you
Every wish that I wish for, is for our love to remain strong
And for every waking day together I want you to know
That is where we belong

For all the up's and downs, for all joys and sadness
For every laugh we share together and for every tear that we should cry
If we do it together then this life should promise us no more goodbyes
And in each other's lives we shall remain forever and ever

Although we shall often find that we do not understand each other
And for this may lead us only to each other to be unkind
If you sit back and close you're eyes and take a deep breath
You shall see our visions of each other
Then only happiness you shall find

So even when the odds are stacked against us
Together we should fight back
Ignore all fears and doubts we have
Then renounce all bad thoughts and forget all that used to be sad

Journey Into My Life

Look to tomorrow and let yesterday remain in the past
And then if we should ever be drawn apart
For every breath I take with you, will allow you to venture down deep into my heart

Now let's not worry for the things that we have done
And think only of the things we want to do
For our time on this earth is too short to waste
And every hatred word spoken and every cry that we cry
Is just another breath wasted of what's left of this precious life

For now and forever my heart is filled with only love for you
For you have become my oxygen supply and so if we should ever part
Failure to breathe leads only to die.

Dated: 4th May

Lisa Diallo

Sitting Alone

Sitting alone with thoughts in my mind
Looking and searching but never to find
The questions all there but no answers to reply
But to myself bad thoughts I can deny

All on my own with nothing to say
Wondering whether I will survive another day
I reach out for someone, someone who cares
My arms are empty as usual, there's nobody there

No one to cry with and no one to laugh with
And no one to take away the pain
I need some guidance through this time
To keep my mind sane

And as I lay my head to sleep and turn out the lights
There's no one who cares to squeeze and hold me tight
But as dawn breaks and the birds sing
I start my day again
And all my thoughts and worries have gone away
And I know that it's time to carry on.

Dated: 20th February 1992

Journey Into My Life

Mixed Signals

I pray do tell me, what is it you're scared of?
Tell me your fears, answer me please
Why is it you push me away?
Every time that I get near

Why is it you act like you don't care?
Always resulting in me feeling that you're being unfair
Yet on the other hand we lay together you some how make everything alright
Resistance then becomes low and the feelings you can no longer fight

And so as the night draws near and I feel your warm embrace
And you pull me so tight
Followed by your gentle touch and your sweet caress
And again you make everything so right

And then so as each other bodies and minds we begin to explore
Brings feelings of passion and longing for more
And it's at these times when I feel there's something there
And all climaxes are reached all emotions explored
Feelings of contentment a reminder that you are
'The one I adore'

Never wanting these feelings to come to an end
Hoping that all bridges we can now mend

Lisa Diallo

For wanting to be your lover and also your best
friend
And then yet again as another day does start
Again re appear those doubts
And these mixed emotions are wiping me out

Back to the unknown wondering
If you shall stay or are just going with the flow
And hoping you never leave me, praying that you
never go.

Dated: 6th October 2006

Journey Into My Life

Who Cares

So now you think you are funny
Well now your fun and games are all done
Because now I have had just about enough
It's over, zero out yes we're done

A friend did say that our move would make or break
us
Looks like the break became favourite
Yes the odds were stacked against
Sick of all your silence when you choose
Your moods you have for no reason
And you do what the hell you like
Well babe I'm sorry to say you just had your last
ride on this bike

Because what is good for you is good for me
And yet again it all just becomes a battle of the
wars
Now I am beginning to realise that this relationship
and so called marriage
All along has been for nothing it has proved to be a
lost cause

Everyone has a breaking point
And now that I have reached mine
Now that I see the light only to realise we have
nothing in common
I guess we never had, I think I just woke up and
smelt the coffee and realised
I must have been mad

Lisa Diallo

What's wrong baby? Did I do something wrong?
Or just something you did not like, or maybe just in
your twisted mind
Is again playing games and as the thoughts inside
your head
You still dwell over
Your imagination has gone wild and your ego is
starting to swell

Yet again resulting in thinking only the worst of me
Because I stayed up and talked to an old friend
And I do not see what it matters to you
As civil words never pass between us, not a full
sentence
To each other do we ever send

God only knows where my head has been all this
time
It would have been easier just to have had a lodger
As that's how life is with you
And every one else could see it, laughing because
they all knew
But with all the things occurring right now, I must
admit I don't give a shit
As out of all my problems in life
You matter not one little bit

And so all that is left to summarise is your attitude
stinks
Your morals are all messed up and for all of this
No you are very welcome and as for you
I don't really give a shit.

Dated: 16th July 2004

Journey Into My Life

Anger

So much anger I feel inside, all my tears I am trying to hide
Everything seems such a mess with everything that I do
Everyday is dull and my life always seems blue
I feel friends are not many as I only have few

My head is all torn to pieces, my heart no longer feels
I feel as though this life has dealt me too many raw deals
But upon myself I have brought them and I now see no way out
They call it insecurity yet still this I have to doubt

But when I need somebody, someone who really cares
I turn around to find them, but surprise surprise
There is no one there, why am I so lonely?
Or maybe it is just me, no one ever understands me
I'm not complicated just that no one takes the time to look that deep
For then all my hurt they would see

But I know that everyone expects more no matter what they do
But now I have nothing left to feel
I guess with this life I am finally through.

Dated: November 1998

Lisa Diallo

Through your eyes

Through your eyes I see it all my love, my life
With you I shall never fall
All up's and downs sometimes make me feel like I
want to walk away
Then a small reminder pulls at my heart, and yet
again with you I stay

For times gone quickly, almost two years since we
met
For our first meeting I shall never forget
But never once would I of said that we would
remain together for so long
And that my feelings for you would grow so strong
Yet everyday for me is a reminder that with you is
where I belong
And maybe in years to come
Together we shall look back or just maybe in years
to come
I shall sit and remember how you I do miss

But whatever this life shall bring us, or wherever we
shall go
These few words are just a reminder of how I loved
you so.

Dated: 6th November 2006

Journey Into My Life

Last Laugh

So yet again you think you can mess with my head
Maybe if you sat back and looked at all the things
you have done to me
All the nasty things you have said, and yet
I am still sat with you
What gives you the right to abuse what I say?
And then threaten we are through

After everything that has happened with us I should
have left long ago
But then again like you always said
'How could anyone want me?!'
Those words you can speak to me no more
What all your games are maybe coming to a reality
Now panicking because the rules have changed
You have messed with my head all these months,
and now have the audacity
For me to blame

I was always taught that honesty was the best
policy
And I thought you would respect me more for that
Or maybe your accusations are there just to cover
your own guilt
The easy way now is our marriage to jilt

Well let me tell you something now
You have messed with my head too many times
Always me being accused, I know about your kind
Well believe what you will and do what the hell you
want

But those thoughts in your head will make you risk losing everything
Especially me
And if that's how you want it then that's how it shall be

But just remember those times you walked away before
It was me who was laid crying behind closed doors
But where were you when my marriage felt like my world was falling apart?
Oh pardon me you were in the ritzy
And you claim I'm the one without any heart
So I suggest you take a long look in the mirror and find out
Who you really are before your mind games take one step too far.

Dated: 13th August 2004

Journey Into My Life

Beyond All Control

The smallest of things seems so big
The smallest of things can even bring regret that you exist
Feels like you are on the road of recovery
Heading at last down the right path
Then for no reason at all it's ruined
Why can happiness never last?

Things beyond control, all things that we cannot decide
All kept away somehow from our eyes they hide
And then bang, back to square one is all that we find
Who was the one that decided this life should be so unkind?

I used to think all was karma coming back round
But seems like mine has been round twice
Feels sometimes like opening and closing of a very tight vice
For its left me to believe that all shall not end,
No hope, no visions, no dreams nothing positive left to send

For I feel this wheel of life is forever turning back on its self
Showing no happiness, no promises and no given wealth
All contributing to going bad health
So I adapt to the fact that my life shall continue to be uncertain

Lisa Diallo

And always wait for the bad that follows the good
I wish only now that I had control of my life
But I am shown that I never had any and never
would.

Dated: 26th March 2003

Journey Into My Life

Just Starting Out

Don't you think its how funny how in this life things work out?
As just when I felt like I wanted to end it all and I could not carry on
For my life was filled with doubts
You came along first as a friend always there to lend a hand
And after each meeting there was no pressure and no demands

Then I found myself questioning about what was occurring here
Filled with excitement and mixed emotions, also present a little fear
For right before my very eyes when I was too blind to see
Somehow my heart had already decided that you were the one for me

Yes I had started to fall into that trap
And the reality of it all was such a shock
As after my last relationship on these kind of feelings
I thought I had managed to block

But it was a barrier that you had managed to break through
Just by being you
And all the little things about you I had grown to love

Lisa Diallo

As all of you inside and out is good through and
through
And I was just wondering what good I had done?
To be rewarded with someone like you

For you entered my life so swiftly
And somehow reached down deep in my heart
And although you made it better
Seems like you managed to keep our feelings apart

And now I am proud to say I love you
And every minute we are apart I hate
As this thing we have created was definitely built on
fate
And destiny cannot be changed for that's just the
way life goes
But I hope and believe that deep down that
together for infinity
We shall remain
As you have brought me happiness and took away
the pain.

Dated: December 2006

Journey Into My Life

Fulfilled Fantasies

Two bodies entangled, our legs entwined
All our hidden fantasies now our minds seek to find
Passion all around becomes an explosion of feelings so unreal
Everything now released especially how we feel

The eruption of all emotions
When our bodies begin to wind and grind
As our breathing becomes heavy as ecstasy we reach
Pleasure alone is now what we find
Memories of nights together is left for us to remind

And as the faded sounds of pleasurable moans and cries are nearly to an end
Shyness, embarrassment has erased all doubts
As each others bodies we did explore
And now everything around us we choose to ignore

For now all has been ventured
Yes every inch of our bodies explored all climaxed
Reached and fantasies soared
As we finally come to our peak at last
Fulfilment now together is what we reach.

Dated: 15th November 2004

Lisa Diallo

Me and You Together

Last night I had a dream that me and you were together
Everything was so real I wanted it to last forever
As romantically we walked, you were holding my hand
And even though I'm not sure why, but somehow I was made to understand

And although I could feel your touch as you gently held my hand
Your vision seemed to fade out across the golden sands
Then all of a sudden my joys turned into fears
Feelings of being scared and alone and sad that you were not here
Yet still I continued to search for you
For defeat was never an option as I was positive you I would find
No matter how tired I did get it was thoughts of you alone
That now filled my mind

And as I slowly dragged myself along
So tired and exhausted with the pains of you not being around
And then as I looked behind me, to my surprise
Your vision is now what I found and then came so strongly
Every possible emotion went through me and such a powerful love is what I felt

Journey Into My Life

And as we embraced, it was at that point in your arms I did melt

And then as I awoke from this dream
I tried to make sense of it all, yes tried to figure it all out
A need to know what it did mean
And so the conclusion I arrived at was this;
If you lose sight of what you are aiming for
Or if somehow you feel like you are losing the one and only
The most important thing in your life
It is shown that you must carry on
Even at those times you think you will never survive

And then it led me to believe that this was a message from above
It was to let us know that no matter what does happen to us
Somehow we shall get through all the up's and downs
As I do believe that true love in you is now what I have found
And therefore my promise I give you is that I shall always be around.

Dated: 23rd November 2004

Lisa Diallo

If You

If you saw someone bleeding would you just walk away?
If you saw a hungry child who needed feeding would you leave them to stray?

And if you saw someone with a broken heart
Would you offer words of comfort?
Or would you stand back and watch them fall apart?

I believe your answers to all would be no
As you cannot not stand or even walk away
And leave them and now I ask so...

So why when I am bleeding inside and am hungry for you
And with every beat of my heart
I miss everything we used to do
And why is it that you are never really there
Why stick around when it's obvious that for me you don't care
And please explain it to me how you find it so easy
To turn and walk away
When I sit here with my heart breaking without you
Every single day.

Dated: January 2007

www.ingramcontent.com/pod-product-compliance
Lightning Source LLC
Chambersburg PA
CBHW031159270326
41931CB00006B/329

* 9 7 8 1 8 4 7 4 7 8 5 9 7 *